Advanced Cardiac
Life Support

ADVANCED CARDIAC LIFE SUPPORT

The practical approach

The Advanced Life Support Group

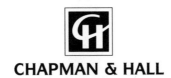

CHAPMAN & HALL

London · Glasgow · New York · Tokyo · Melbourne · Madras

Published by Chapman & Hall, 2-6 Boundary Row, London SE1 8HN

Chapman & Hall, 2-6 Boundary Row, London SE1 8HN, UK

Blackie Academic & Professional, Wester Cleddens Road, Bishopbriggs, Glasgow G64 2NZ, UK

Chapman & Hall, 29 West 35th Street, New York NY10001, USA

Chapman & Hall Japan, Thomson Publishing Japan, Hirakawacho Nemoto Building, 6F, 1-7-11 Hirakawa-cho, Chiyoda-ku, Tokyo 102, Japan

Chapman & Hall Australia, Thomas Nelson Australia, 102 Dodds Street, South Melbourne, Victoria 3205, Australia

Chapman & Hall India, R. Seshadri, 32 Second Main Road, CIT East, Madras 600 035, India

First edition 1993
Reprinted 1993

© 1993 Chapman & Hall

Typeset in 12/14pt Palatino by Columns Design & Production Services Ltd., Reading
Printed in Great Britain by TJ Press Ltd, Padstow, Cornwall

ISBN 0 412 48390 4

A catalogue record for this book is available from the British Library
Library of Congress Cataloging-in-Publication Data available

Contents

List of contributors

Peter Barnes FRCP
Patrick Dando MRCGP
Peter Driscoll FRCS
Gill Ellison SRN
Olive Goodall SRN
Sarah Graham MRCP
Carl Gwinnutt FFARCS
Mark James DA FRCS
Kevin Mackway-Jones MRCP FRCS
Elizabeth Molyneux MRCP
Peter Nightingale MRCP FFARCS
Peter Oakley MA FFARCS
Richard Old
Barbara Phillips FRCP
Brian Reilly
John Shaffer MRCP
Andrew Swain PhD FRCS
Marion Waters FRCS
Susan Wieteska
David Yates MA MD MCh FRCS

Preface

Advanced Cardiac Life Support: The Practical Approach has been written to enable all healthcare workers to manage a cardiac emergency safely and effectively. This manual also forms a part of an integrated learning package aimed at enabling ACLS candidates to complete an ACLS course successfully and gain ACLS provider status. It is not a manual of cardiology or anaesthetics, nor, if read in isolation, does it profess to teach all that is required of the ACLS provider. In particular a manual cannot teach the practical skills that are necessary during resuscitation. Readers who have not attended a course are therefore encouraged to do so.

The text is written with practice in the United Kingdom in mind, and incorporates the recommendations for cardiac arrest treatment provided by the European Resuscitation Council. The style is deliberately didactic, and only generally acceptable and available treatments are included. As practice changes, and newer treatments are accepted, the course will evolve to include them.

ACLS training, of which this manual forms a part, aims to provide a solid and safe foundation of knowledge and skills which can be built on. It does not represent the end of learning.

Editorial Board: P.A. Driscoll, C. Gwinnutt, K. Mackway-Jones, S. Wieteska

Acknowledgements

We are indebted to Mary Harrison MMAA and Keith Harrison AIMBI, MMAA who successfully translated our descriptions into the line diagrams you see in this book.

The faculty also gratefully acknowledges the continued support of Laerdal (UK) Ltd, without whose help this course could not have developed to the degree that it has. In addition Hoechst (UK) Ltd have kindly given permission for Figures 7.15–7.21, 7.23, 7.24, 7.29–7.31, 7.34, 7.37 and 9.13 to be reproduced from their excellent ECG Atlas.

We also wish to thank the ECG Department at Hope Hospital, Salford and the Coronary Care Unit at the University Hospital of South Manchester for providing other ECGs.

The faculty thanks, in retrospect, those candidates who have offered constructive criticism after taking this course, and would like to thank in advance those of you currently taking the course who will no doubt also have useful suggestions.

Appendix B, 'Ethical and legal considerations in resuscitation', by Dr Patrick Dando, was first published as 'Medico-legal problems associated with resuscitation' in the *Journal of the Medical Defence Union*, Volume 8, Numbers 1 and 2, 1992. It is reproduced here with kind permission of the Medical Defence Union and Dr Patrick Dando. All rights reserved.

Objectives for an ACLS provider

To know the essential core content described in the manual:

Relevant pathophysiology
Dysrhythmia recognition
Immediate and advanced treatment of a cardiac emergency
Relevant post-resuscitation care

To have the practical skills to carry out safely and effectively:

Basic cardiac life support
Basic and advanced airway management
Defibrillation and monitoring
Vascular access

To have the ability to:

Lead a cardiac resuscitation
Be an effective member of the resuscitation team

—— 1 ——
Introduction

Objectives

After studying this chapter you should be able to:

- Understand the aims of the manual
- Understand the history of advanced cardiac life support
- Give an overview of:

  The epidemiology and aetiology of heart disease
  The pathophysiology of heart disease
  The activities required in managing a cardiac arrest

1.1 THE AIMS OF THE MANUAL

There are many ways of managing a cardiac emergency. This manual aims to teach a system which is known to be both safe and effective. It will **not** train readers to be cardiologists or anaesthetists, but it will enable them to deal with a cardiac emergency in a logical and systematic way, thereby facilitating later management by other medical specialists.

1.2 THE HISTORY OF ADVANCED CARDIAC LIFE SUPPORT

In 1973 an advanced cardiac life support (ACLS) package was produced by the American Heart Association. This was subsequently updated in 1980 and 1985 to incorporate new information and changes in practice. Eighteen years on, tens of thousands of health care providers have successfully completed the ACLS course.

In 1987, the Royal College of Physicians published a report advocating the need for both basic and advanced life support training in health care providers [1]. In the same year, David Skinner set up the UK's first American-style ACLS course at St Bartholomew's Hospital, London. Since then, several centres have run courses, with various standards being taught.

In 1990 a group of clinicians from five acute specialities, along with an educationalist, developed the course of which this manual forms a part. It was based upon the US course but modified to account for European clinicians and their way of practice. In particular, the guidelines from the Resuscitation Council (UK) were incorporated.

Material is presented in a didactic fashion. Some of the latest therapeutic programmes and concepts have not been included, either because they are not universally available, or because they are not generally accepted. In the future, the course content will evolve as treatments and techniques are modified and are agreed.

The authors have also taken into account the feedback from doctors, nurses and paramedics who have now completed this course. The end result is a tried and tested educational package, which is relevant for all health care personnel working in the acute sector.

It is important to realize that the knowledge gained is aimed at enhancing, not replacing, the in-house training personnel already received in their own hospitals or institutions.

1.3 AN OVERVIEW OF THE EPIDEMIOLOGY AND AETIOLOGY OF HEART DISEASE

The sudden cardiac event known as a cardiac arrest is usually the end stage of a long pathological process. In 80% of cases the patient is known to have heart disease, but in the remaining 20% a cardiac arrest is the first clinical presentation.

There are many contributory factors, but ischaemic heart disease is by far the most common. In the UK, this leads to approximately 500/100 000 deaths a year in male and female patients aged between 45 and 69 years. These figures are among the highest in the world.

The American experience indicates that preventative methods can reduce the incidence of death due to cardiovascular disease. Consequently, the development of advanced life support techniques should not be viewed as an excuse to continue unhealthy diets and life styles. Prevention is more effective, and much cheaper, than the present day cure.

1.4 AN OVERVIEW OF THE PATHOPHYSIOLOGY OF HEART DISEASE

Many factors can act on the myocardium to produce an abnormal cardiac function (Figure 1.1).

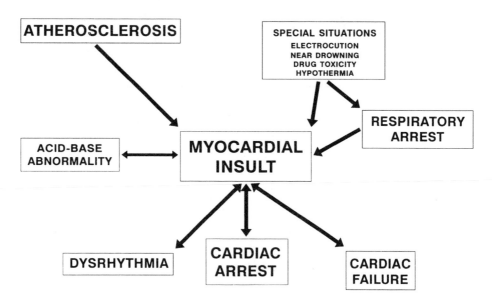

Fig. 1.1 Aetiologies of myocardial damage

This may or may not involve death of the actual muscle. In certain cases, the causative factors also affect other sites in the body. In most cases, several of these factors are acting concurrently.

The resuscitation team has to be aware of these causative factors and each of their potential end results, so that the correct treatment can be provided.

1.5 THE ACTIVITIES REQUIRED IN MANAGING A CARDIAC ARREST

The majority of cardiac arrests occur outside hospital. Therefore, in order for the patient to survive, a whole series of activities needs to be carried out quickly, effectively and in the correct order:

1. Recognition
2. Commencement of basic life support techniques
3. Defibrillation
4. Advanced life support techniques
5. Post-resuscitation care
6. Rehabilitation

Studies by Eisenberg *et al.* in Seattle [2], have shown that the patient's eventual outcome is very dependent on the speed of onset and the efficiency of the basic and advanced life support techniques (Table 1.1).

Table 1.1 Incidence of survival following basic and advanced CPR [2]

Time to CPR (min)	Time to ACLS (min)		
	<8	8–16	>16
0–4	43%	19%	10%
4–8	26%	19%	5%
8–12		6%	0%

It follows that ACLS is only going to be of use if effective community cardiopulmonary resuscitation (CPR) can be carried out quickly, and the patient can be defibrillated rapidly. Many reports have demonstrated how successful early defibrillation can be.

The authors hope that readers of this manual will become involved in teaching and organizing their own community CPR programmes. In that way the skills discussed can be used to greater effect.

REFERENCES

1. Royal College of Physicians (1987) Resuscitation from cardiopulmonary arrest: training and organisation. *J. R. Coll. Physicians (Lond.)*, **21**, 1.

2. Eisenberg, M., Bergner, L. and Hallstrom, A. (1979) Cardiac resuscitation in the community. Importance of rapid provision and implications for programme planning. *J. Am. Med. Assoc.*, **241**, 1905.

2
Basic life support

Objectives

After studying this chapter you should be able to:

- Understand the basic support of airway, breathing and circulation
- Demonstrate to a satisfactory standard the basic life support of a collapsed patient

2.1 INTRODUCTION

Basic life support (BLS) means maintaining an airway and supporting breathing and circulation in anyone who is in need of such help **without any equipment**. No consideration of advanced cardiac life support (ACLS) techniques in children and adults can begin without the preliminary acquisition of BLS skills.

This chapter will concentrate on the principles of BLS and its practice in adults. Paediatric BLS will be discussed in detail in Chapter 9.

Survival from cardiac arrest is more likely when the arrest is witnessed, and bystander resuscitation is commenced. Studies have indicated that survival rates are improved when time from collapse to initiation of BLS is short. Furthermore, the speed of initiation of BLS may be more important than the absolute quality of the technique employed. However, BLS must be started early and continued during advanced life support procedures.

In general, BLS should be started in all patients who suddenly become unresponsive and who are either apnoeic or have an absent major pulse (carotid or femoral). If cardiac arrest occurs in hospital and an up-to-date, signed 'Not for Resuscitation' order is in force this is inappropriate.

2.2 THE SAFE APPROACH

Assessment should begin as soon as possible after the collapse occurs or the patient is found. However, the rescuer must not become a second victim, and further harm to the patient must be avoided. Thus, prior to assessing the condition of the patient the rescuer should **S**hout, to summon help, **A**pproach the patient with care, **F**ree the patient from any continuing danger before **E**valuating the airway, breathing and circulation (ABC). This is summarized in Figure 2.1.

Shout for help

Approach with care

Free from danger

Evaluate ABC

Fig. 2.1   The SAFE approach

Unresponsiveness is assessed by asking the patient "Are you all right?" and **gently** shaking them by the shoulder.

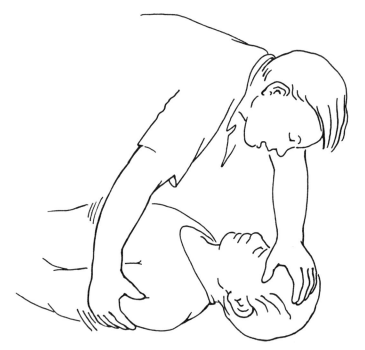

Fig. 2.2   "Are you all right?"

Remember that in cases associated with trauma the neck and spine should be protected by immobilizing the head during this manoeuvre (the head is firmly held with one hand flat on the forehead and one arm is gently shaken; Figure 2.2). If the patient responds by answering or moving, they should not be moved unless they are not safe. Remember that they may deteriorate, so they must be reassessed and help should be called for if needed.

If there is no response to voice or touch, help should be called for again if none has arrived.

In the spontaneously breathing patient who has suffered trauma, the cervical spine can be protected by in-line cervical stabilization. This technique is shown in Figure 2.3.

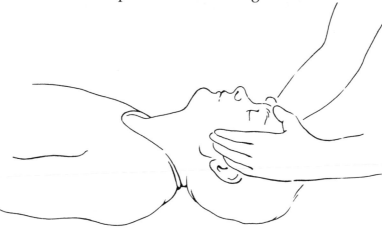

Fig. 2.3 In-line cervical stabilization

2.3 THE ABCs

2.3.1 Airway

An obstructed airway may be the primary problem and correction of this may achieve recovery without further intervention. This is most often caused by the relaxed tongue falling backwards onto the posterior wall of the pharynx.

The primary method of attaining an airway is by using the head tilt/chin lift technique (Figure 2.4).

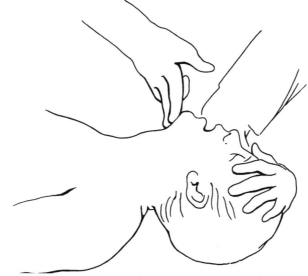

Fig. 2.4 Head tilt/ chin lift

The rescuer places the hand nearest to the victim's head on the forehead, and gently tilts the head back. The fingers of the other hand are placed under the chin, and the jaw is lifted upwards. As this may cause the mouth to close, it may be necessary to use the thumb to part the lips. The success of this manoeuvre should be assessed immediately by looking, listening and feeling.

Looking: to see if the chest is rising and falling
Listening: to hear any breathing or gurgling/snoring sounds
Feeling: with the cheek near the victim's mouth for exhaled breath or with the hand on the chest for movement

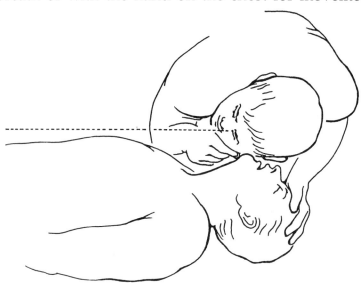

Fig. 2.5 Look, listen and feel technique

If head tilt/chin lift is not appropriate, two other techniques can be tried. First, if foreign material may be obstructing the airway, attempts should be made to remove this using a finger sweep (Figure 2.6).

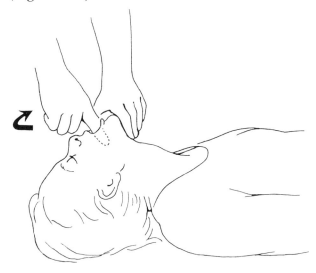

Fig. 2.6 Finger sweep

The mouth is opened and inspected, and two fingers are gently swept from the side to the back. If any debris is found attempts should be made to hook it out. Loose or broken dentures should be removed at this stage.

The jaw thrust may also be used to move the tongue forward (Figure 2.7).

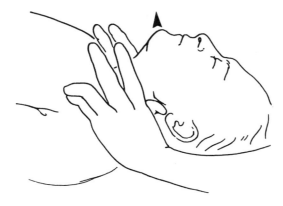

Fig. 2.7 Jaw thrust

Two fingers or the thumbs of the rescuer's hands are placed behind each angle of the victim's mandible. The mandible is then thrust anteriorly. The jaw thrust **alone** should be used to open the airway if an injury to the cervical spine is suspected.

The results of these manoeuvres should be assessed by looking, listening and feeling.

The above sequence should be performed rapidly.

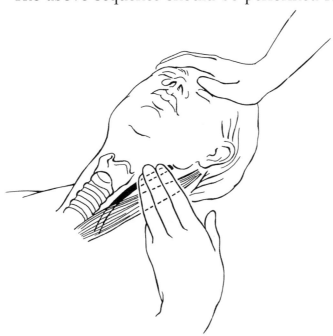

Fig.2.8 Feeling for the carotid pulse

A major pulse should be felt for (e.g. carotid or femoral, Figure 2.8).

The radial pulse is **not** satisfactory as it may be absent in otherwise normal patients. The pulse must be sought for at least 5 s to make sure there is no circulation.

2.3.2 Breathing

The patient may start to breathe after the simple airway manoeuvres carried out during assessment. If this occurs they should be placed in the recovery position and help should be sought immediately.

9

If the patient is not breathing and a pulse **is** present, then 10 rescue breaths must be given before help is sought.

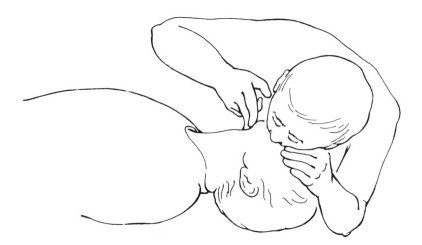

**Fig. 2.9
Expired air
resuscitation**

To perform expired air resuscitation effectively (Figure 2.9), there should be no obstruction or leakage to airflow between the rescuer and the patient's lungs. This is best achieved by placing the flat of the uppermost hand on the victim's forehead, tilting the head and using the fingers of that hand to pinch the patient's nose shut. The other hand is used to lift the chin forward and open the mouth.

The rescuer takes a deep breath, seals their lips round those of the victim and breathes out into their mouth, watching to ensure that the chest rises. Well-fitting dentures can be left in place as it can be very difficult to get a good seal in an edentulous patient. Loose or broken dentures should be removed. If the chest does not rise, either the airway may not be fully open or the seal may be inadequate. After each breath the victim should be allowed to exhale passively to the atmosphere.

Mouth to mouth and nose ventilation can be used in children and may be appropriate in water rescue. In these cases the mouth must be opened to allow expiration.

Mouth to mask ventilation using a portable face-mask is also recommended as a suitable technique, but rescue breathing should not be delayed if this device is not available.

Each rescue breath should last 1½–2 s. Following this 2–4 s should be allowed for expiration.

2.3.3 Circulation

2.3.3.1 Assessment

If the patient is apnoeic and pulseless help should be sought immediately. Once this has been done full CPR should be started.

2.3.3.2 External cardiac compression

To generate an optimum cardiac output, the position of the hands is very important – if they are too high the efficiency of cardiopulmonary resuscitation (CPR) is reduced and if too low the stomach is compressed and aspiration becomes more likely. In an adult the correct hand placement for external massage is two finger breadths above the xiphisternum (Figure 2.10).

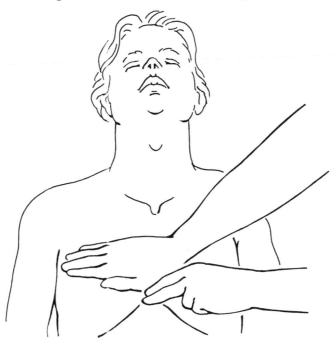

**Fig. 2.10
Landmarks for
adult cardiac
compressions**

The rescuer must carefully reposition their hands after each interruption in cardiac compression. The heel of one hand is placed over the correct part of the sternum and the other hand is placed on top of it with the fingers interlocked (Figure 2.11).

In order to compress the chest wall downwards the rescuer must have sufficient height above the patient for their hands, elbows and shoulders to extend down in a vertical line. If the patient is on a trolley, a stool or special CPR bar may be used to achieve this. Sternal depression of 4–5 cm is said to be ideal in an adult. Optimum compression, with minimum rescuer fatigue, can be achieved by keeping the arms straight and leaning forwards. This transmits the rescuer's body weight to the patient's chest. Flexing the elbows and pumping the arms up and down may achieve adequate compressions in the short term, but fatigue in the rescuer will soon reduce their efficiency.

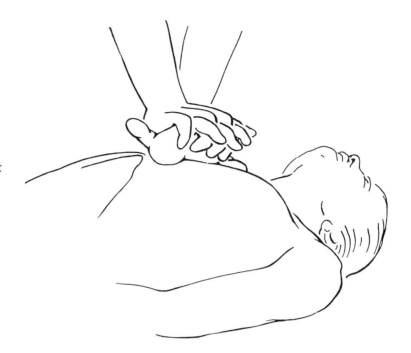

Fig. 2.11 Hand position for adult cardiac compressions

Cardiac compressions should be applied at a rate of 60–80 per min. The rate can be controlled by counting aloud 'one and two and three . . .'.

If a single rescuer is present and the patient is an adult then two breaths should be delivered, followed by 15 compressions. Two rescuers should provide compressions and breaths in a ratio of 5:1 (Figure 2.12).

Fig. 2.12 Two-rescuer technique

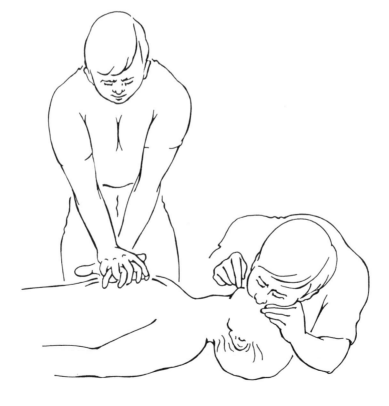

BLS must not be interrupted unless the patient starts to move or breathe spontaneously.

2.4 SUMMARY OF BLS SEQUENCE

The sequence of BLS in cardiopulmonary arrest is summarised in Figure 2.13.

Fig. 2.13 The sequence of basic life support in cardiopulmonary arrest

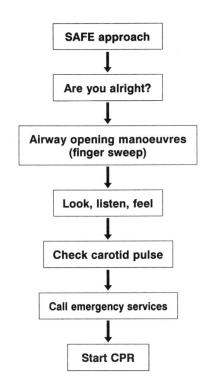

SAFE approach

↓

Are you alright?

↓

Airway opening manoeuvres
(finger sweep)

↓

Look, listen, feel

↓

Check carotid pulse

↓

Call emergency services

↓

Start CPR

2.5 RECOVERY

If the patient starts to breathe spontaneously he/she should be turned into the recovery position and the open airway maintained (Figure 2.14).

Fig. 2.14 Recovery position

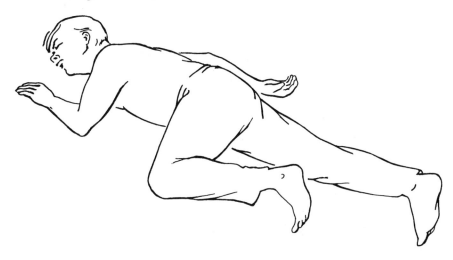

This position will allow vomit to dribble out rather than be aspirated and obstruct the airway. The tongue will not fall backwards and obstruct the airway in this position. Note that if spinal injury is suspected the patient should not be moved until five people are available to log-roll the patient into the spinal recovery position.

2.6 THE CHOKING PATIENT

Almost any foreign body can obstruct the airway. The commonest situation in healthy adults is the 'cafe coronary', in which food is inhaled, usually because of an attempt to talk, drink and eat simultaneously. People with an impaired 'gag' reflex and the elderly are also prone to choking.

Recognition is of prime importance. There is sudden loss of airway patency, usually accompanied by vigorous attempts to dislodge the obstruction. Patients with partial obstruction may cough and have inspiratory stridor. Any patient who suddenly shows signs of airway obstruction should be assumed to be choking.

Vigorous back blows can sometimes be curative. If not, the Heimlich manoeuvre should be performed (Figure 2.15).

Fig. 2.15 Heimlich manoeuvre

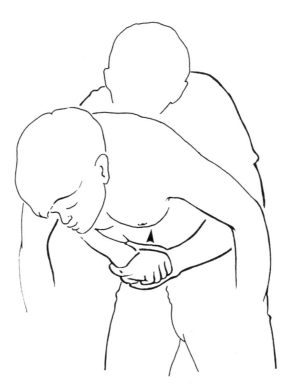

This manoeuvre, which can be carried out with the patient standing, sitting, kneeling or lying (if unconscious), is an attempt to expel the foreign body by increasing intrathoracic pressure by forcing the diaphragm upwards into the chest. Unless the patient is lying down, the rescuer should move behind them. The rescuer's arms are passed around the victim, and one hand is formed into a fist and placed in the epigastrium. The other hand is placed over the fist and both are forced vigorously upwards. This should be repeated 5–10 times unless the obstruction is relieved sooner. If the victim is unconscious they should be placed supine so that the rescuer can kneel astride them and place their hands on the abdomen as described above. In this situation care should be taken to direct the abdominal thrusts in the midline (Figure 2.16).

**Fig. 2.16
Abdominal thrusts**

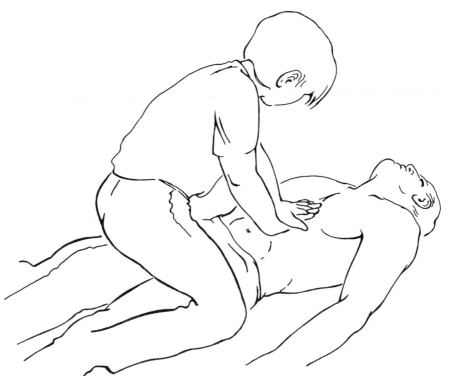

If the foreign body is not expelled at the first attempt, then a further two series of 10 thrusts should be performed. In the pre-hospital situation there is little else that can be done unless a skilled person capable of surgical airway management is present.

2.7 BLS: TRAINING AND DECAY OF SKILLS

Many studies show that BLS skills decay very quickly when not used on a regular basis. Therefore practical training and regular updating are essential if acceptable standards are to be achieved and maintained.

Practical skill station
Basic life support

AIMS

To reinforce practically the basic life support procedures demonstrated during the theoretical sessions.

To allow candidates to demonstrate proficiency in basic life support procedures.

TEACHING TECHNIQUE

Basic life support procedures are revised and practised using a basic life support manikin.

TESTING

Candidates are assessed practically using a basic life support manikin and monitor.

3

The natural history of myocardial infarction

Objectives

After studying this chapter you should be able to:

- Understand the epidemiology and pathogenesis of myocardial infarction

- Understand how to recognize myocardial infarction clinically

- Understand the immediate management of myocardial infarction

3.1 EPIDEMIOLOGY OF ISCHAEMIC HEART DISEASE

The term 'ischaemic heart disease' (IHD) covers a wide variety of syndromes from silent myocardial ischaemia to sudden cardiac death encompassing angina pectoris and myocardial infarction (MI). The common underlying pathology is atheroma of the coronary arteries. Mortality rates for IHD in the United Kingdom are among the highest in the world at approximately 500/100 000 for men and women aged 40–69. There are clearly declining trends, however, and in England and Wales for men aged 50–59 the IHD death rate in 1985 was about 25% less than in 1975. Similar trends are present in women, those aged 40–49 showing the most marked decline in the past decade.

Risk factors for the presence of IHD include:

Increasing age
Male sex
Cigarette smoking
Family history
Hypertension
Serum cholesterol

3.2 PATHOGENESIS

Arteriosclerosis is a slowly progressive focal proliferation of connective tissue within the intima. These changes can be seen in adolescence. Interstitial proliferation (leading to segmental narrowing of the coronary arteries to an extent that there is flow-limitation on exercise) causes typical stable angina. Sudden thrombosis at the site of an atheromatous plaque is responsible for the acute presentations of IHD, including unstable angina, MI and sudden death. Plaque fissuring is responsible for the majority of major thrombi. A tear extends from the lumen through the intima into the plaque and the entry of blood provokes the formation of a platelet-dominated thrombus within the intima. A small proportion progress to the formation of an overlying intraluminal thrombus. Many factors determine whether or not intraluminal thrombus develops, including the coagulability of the blood at the time and the size of the tear.

3.3 ACUTE MYOCARDIAL INFARCTION

Acute myocardial infarction is defined as myocardial necrosis due to cessation or interference with the blood supply. Histologically recognizable changes do not develop for 6–8 h; thus patients dying suddenly will not have enzymatic or morphological evidence of infarction. Macroscopic infarct may be regional when it is related to thrombosis in the supplying artery, or diffuse when it reflects an overall fall in myocardial perfusion (as in extensive atheromatous disease or in cardiogenic shock following a regional infarction).

3.4 PROGNOSIS OF A MYOCARDIAL INFARCTION

At the onset of symptoms of a heart attack the prognosis is bad, with 50% of patients dying. Myocardial rupture can occur within a few hours and ventricular dysrhythmias (which bear no relation to the size of the infarct) also occur very early. Consequently, 60% of deaths from MI occur within the first 2–3 h. For those reaching hospital and receiving appropriate treatment the mortality rate approximates to 10%. For those surviving 1 year the annual fatality rate is about 5%.

High risk groups can be identified by clinical assessment and investigation, and referred for coronary artery surgery.

3.5 CLINICAL RECOGNITION AND IMMEDIATE CARE OF MYOCARDIAL INFARCTION

MI may occur silently or present with complications such as rhythm disturbances, but the overwhelming majority of patients give a history of severe persistent chest pain. Its characteristics and radiations are well known. It is worth emphasizing that occurrence of pain at a remote site, e.g. the wrist, without pain also being present in the chest is unusual. Commonly, there are no abnormal physical findings relating to the cardiovascular systems; the most consistent finding is evidence of autonomic activity with sweating, tachycardia, pallor and peripheral vaso-constriction. Vagal influences occasionally dominate the picture with bradycardia and nausea.

3.5.1 Confirmation and diagnosis

Electrocardiography is invaluable in the diagnosis of MI and should be performed immediately in all suspected cases. It is essential to recognize, however, that a normal cardiograph early in the evolution of the illness does not exclude the diagnosis. If the clinical circumstances strongly suggest MI, management decisions should not be delayed pending cardiographic change.

Cardiac enzymes are only useful in confirming the diagnosis retrospectively. Even the rapid rise of creatinine phosphokinase (CPK) does not occur early enough for intervention to be deferred until the result is available.

3.5.2 Immediate care of the patient with myocardial infarction

At the onset of symptoms the patient is at high risk and usually in pain. Resuscitation facilities must be at hand as soon as possible. The patient should be transferred to hospital, paramedical staff with defibrillators or mobile coronary care units being used if immediately available.

A GTN tablet or two puffs from a GTN spray should be given if not already taken by the patient. Oxygen should be given if available.

If pain persists for more than a few minutes opiate analgesia should be given. It is almost always necessary. An injection of 2.5–10 mg of diamorphine should be given intravenously, preferably through an IV cannula. This will need to be accompanied by an anti-emetic, e.g. prochlorperazine 12.5 mg IM. The dose of analgesia should be titrated against the patient's pain.

19

3.6 MYOCARDIAL SALVAGE

3.6.1 Thrombolysis

Early use of aspirin and of thrombolytics has been shown to reduce mortality in acute MI.

Intravenous streptokinase has been shown to be effective in dissolving an intracoronary thrombus in 45%–75% of patients and reduces myocardial damage. It also reduces 1 year mortality by 15%–20%. Aspirin given at the same time appears to have additional benefit and both should be given unless contraindicated.

Tissue plasminogen activator (rT-PA) and anisoylated plasminogen streptokinase activator complex (Apsac) have also been shown to be effective, but recent trials have shown no significant difference between them in terms of reduced mortality. At present streptokinase is the thrombolytic agent of choice and should be given to all patients with suspected or definite MI if the onset is within 24 h and when there are no known contraindications.

Contraindications include:

1. Previous streptokinase in the period more than 5 days and less than 12 months ago.
2. Known allergy to streptokinase or anistreplase (Apsac)
3. Systolic BP less than 90 mmHg.

In these situations rT-PA should be used.

MI in the elderly is more common and produces a higher mortality than in younger patients. Although the risk of bleeding is higher, the risk–benefit analysis for thrombolytic therapy is more favourable and age *per se* is not a contraindication to treatment.

3.6.2 Beta-blockers

The ISIS 1 study suggested IV atenolol given immediately after a patient's admission with MI and followed by one week of oral therapy reduces mortality by 15%. It may prevent one cardiac arrest, one re-infarction and one death in approximately every 200 patients treated. The improved survival is largely achieved by preventing death from acute cardiac rupture within the first 24 h. In general, acute beta-blockade should be avoided in patients with bradycardia, heart failure and hypotension, but is particularly useful in patients with persistent pain, hypertension or inappropriate tachycardia.

3.6.3 Nitrates

Intravenous nitrates given early after the onset of symptoms probably reduce mortality. This could be due to reduction in infarct size by the reversal of an associated element of spasm even in thrombotic coronary occlusion. The role of oral or sublingual nitrates in relation to thrombolytic therapy is yet to be determined, but it seems appropriate to give nitrates by a sublingual preparation as a first-aid measure.

3.7 DYSRHYTHMIAS

Ventricular fibrillation (VF) is most likely to occur with the onset of coronary occlusion. The risks diminish rapidly with time so that safe arrival at hospital is a genuinely reassuring event. Primary VF is unrelated to the size of the infarct and so-called herald arrhythmias are rarely observed. Large infarcts with a correspondingly poor prognosis predispose to late VF, but there is little evidence that 'secondary prevention' with anti-arrhythmics is beneficial.

It is usual to follow successful defibrillation with IV lignocaine as a bolus of 50–100 mg. This is followed by an infusion of 4 mg/min for 30 min with a progressive reduction to 2 mg/min, the infusion being continued for 24–36 h. If defibrillation occurred within the first 12 h no follow-up oral medication is needed. If VF is late or recurrent, oral anti-arrhythmics are given after the standard management of VF. It is not yet clear how long the treatment should be given for or, indeed, whether the benefits of treatment outweigh the risks.

Ventricular tachycardia (VT) (greater than 120 beats/min) is usually associated with large infarcts. It should be treated, and IV lignocaine is the drug of choice if the patient has no symptoms and signs. If successful, this may be followed by oral anti-arrhythmics. If these are unsuccessful or there is immediate haemodynamic deterioration elective cardioversion is preferable.

Idioventricular rhythm ('slow ventricular tachycardia', less than 120 beats/min) and ventricular ectopic beats do not require treatment. The patients' electrolytes should be reviewed to exclude hypokalaemia.

Atrial fibrillation (AF) is often self-limiting and, if the patient is well, even digoxin may not be necessary. If haemodynamic consequences are apparent elective cardioversion should be considered.

Supraventricular tachycardias (SVT) are uncommon in MI. The management of these is as that described in Chapter 8.

Bradycardias and A-V blocks are most common with inferior infarctions. The management of these is as that described in Chapter 8.

3.8 CARDIAC FAILURE

Heart failure is more common after anterior infarction and should be treated along conventional lines. Heart failure may be severe with second or subsequent infarcts whatever the site. The likelihood of heart failure is reduced after successful thrombolysis. It is important to recognize and treat arrhythmias which may have precipitated the failure.

In patients with inferior infarction who have heart failure without pulmonary oedema the possibility of right ventricular infarction should be considered. Such patients are made worse by diuretics and may require intravenous fluids. Pulmonary artery wedge pressure measurements are necessary under these circumstances to monitor progress.

3.9 PSYCHOLOGICAL ASPECTS OF MYOCARDIAL INFARCTION

The psychological impact of MI upon the patient and relatives is very high. Anxiety and chest pain both increase catecholamine levels and increase the risk of rhythm disturbance. Reassurance and analgesia are both important – remember that a patient on admission has already survived the period of greatest risk. Reassurance is enhanced by an air of quiet confidence among the medical attendants.

Under ideal circumstances all patients with suspected MI would be admitted immediately to a Coronary Care Unit (CCU). This is unlikely ever to be achieved and important aspects of initial management are likely to occur outside hospital, in the Accident and Emergency department and in the Intensive Care Unit (ICU). Lack of communication is often a problem and seriously undermines patients' and relatives' confidence. Close liaison between all people involved in the patient's management is essential. The initial management of the patient should be seen as the first step in the process of rehabilitation.

4

Pharmacology

Objectives

After studying this chapter you should be able to:

- Understand the actions, indications and dosages of drugs used in cardiac resuscitation

- Understand the special precautions and contraindications for drugs used in cardiac resuscitation

- Given a simulated patient model, demonstrate the correct prescriptions of drugs in cardiac arrest rhythms, tachyarrhythmias and bradyarrhythmias

4.1 INTRODUCTION

This chapter discusses drugs used in cardiac arrest and dysrhythmias. There are some specialized drugs mentioned in Chapters 9 and 10 which are described in context. They are laid out alphabetically in the main part of this chapter.

4.1.1 Cardiac arrest drugs

The following are covered in this chapter:

Adrenaline
Atropine
Bretylium
Calcium
Lignocaine
Sodium bicarbonate

4.1.2 Drugs used in arrhythmias

The following are covered in this chapter:

Adenosine
Amiodarone
Atenolol (see beta-blockers)
Beta-blockers

Digoxin
Isoprenaline
Verapamil

The Vaughan–Williams classification of anti-arrhythmic agents is used. This is shown in Table 4.1.

Table 4.1 Classification of anti-arrhythmic drugs according to their mechanism of action

Class	Action
I	'Local anaesthetic' drugs which diminish membrane responsiveness and conductivity by reducing sodium ion flux into the cells
IA	Usually prolong repolarization
IB	Usually shorten repolarization
IC	Little effect on repolarization
II	Antagonize the effects of catecholamines without direct effects on cardiac tissue β adrenergic blockade
III	Prolong the action potential without affecting membrane responsiveness
IV	Calcium channel blockade

If a drug can **treat** arrhythmias it can **cause** arrhythmias.

4.1.3 Other drugs

The following are covered in this chapter:

Aspirin
Diazepam
Inotropic agents
Naloxone
Nitrates
Opiates
Thrombolytics

4.2 INDIVIDUAL DRUGS

4.2.1 Adenosine

Indications for use:
Supraventricular tachycardia (SVT)
Undiagnosed wide complex tachycardia

The dose is 6 mg, given rapidly by injection into a large vein, followed by a saline flush. The injection must be fast to achieve adequate and effective blood levels, as the half-life is only 10–15 s.

Adenosine should only be used in a monitored environment, e.g. Coronary Care Unit (CCU), Intensive Care Unit (ICU) or Accident and Emergency Department.

Adenosine is a naturally occurring purine nucleotide. It is a class IV anti-arrhythmic agent. It slows conduction across the atrio-ventricular (A-V) node but has little effect on other myocardial cells.

Administration of adenosine is associated with a wide variety of 'strange feelings' which may include severe chest pain. Patients should be warned to expect these, and reassured that they will settle very quickly without further treatment. This drug may also induce or worsen bronchospasm but only in patients who have asthma. It is antagonized by theophylline. Although adenosine is very effective in terminating an SVT, the short duration of action means that this dysrhythmia could start again. It has no effect on atrial fibrillation or flutter. The major advantage of adenosine is that, unlike verapamil, it can be given to a patient with a broad complex tachycardia of uncertain aetiology. An SVT will be terminated, but a ventricular tachycardia (VT) will continue unchanged, and without significant negative inotropic effects, i.e. any decrease in ventricular contractility resulting in decreased cardiac output and blood pressure. Adenosine can also be given safely to a patient who is on beta-blockers.

4.2.2 Adrenaline

Indications for use:
Preservation of cerebral blood flow in all types of cardiac arrest. (First drug in each of the cardiac arrest protocols.)

In cardiac arrest, the intravenous dose is 1 mg initially, or 2–3 mg via the endotracheal tube (where appropriate, and where venous access is delayed or cannot be achieved). 3 mg may be given as a fourth dose in EMD or asystole.

Adrenaline is a naturally occurring catecholamine which acts as a neurotransmitter in the sympathetic nervous system. It has β_1 and β_2 agonist effects, which result in increased heart rate (chronotropic effect), increased force of contraction (inotropic effect) and bronchodilatation. It has α agonist activity which leads to an increase in the peripheral vascular resistance. This tends to 'divert' blood flow to the brain and heart in the cardiac arrest situation.

Adrenaline is available in two dilutions, 1 in 10 000 (1 g in 10 000 ml) and 1 in 1000 (1 g in 1000 ml). Thus 1 mg = 1 ml of 1:1000 = 10 ml of 1:10 000.

In cardiac resuscitation, the 1 in 10 000 dilution is used, and the 1 mg dose is repeated every 2–3 min until resuscitation is successful or abandoned. The paediatric dose is 10 µg/kg (= 0.01 mg/kg). Adrenaline increases myocardial excitability, and is arrhythmogenic, especially to an ischaemic or hypoxic myocardium, but these effects are not relevant to the cardiac arrest situation or immediate post-resuscitation care.

4.2.3 Amiodarone

Indications for use:
All resistant arrhythmias including VF
Wolfe–Parkinson–White syndrome

A loading dose of 5 mg/kg in 100 ml 5% dextrose (not saline) is given over 1–4 h. The maximum dose is 1.2 g in 24 h. There is a latent period of some hours before the onset of full action. It can then be given orally for 5–10 days, e.g. 200 mg daily.

Amiodarone is classified as a class III anti-arrhythmic agent because it increases the duration of the action potential and therefore the QT interval. It also has some class I activity, inhibiting fast sodium channels. When given IV, it has some non-competitive α-blocking effects. It has a mild negative inotropic effect and is also a coronary artery vasodilator.

If given concurrently with other drugs which act to prolong the QT interval, amiodarone may 'paradoxically' become pro-arrhythmogenic.

If the patient is on warfarin or digoxin, when amiodarone is introduced, the doses of the former should be halved. Amiodarone may react adversely with beta-blockers or verapamil, causing an increased degree of nodal block.

Most of the side effects of amiodarone are not relevant to emergency treatment, although nausea is common, even at low doses. Other side effects occur after prolonged administration, e.g. photosensitive 'blue' skin discolouration, abnormalities of thyroid function, corneal microdeposits and pulmonary infiltrates.

4.2.4 Aspirin

Indications for use:
Anti-thrombotic effect, post-myocardial infarction
Unstable angina to prevent infarction
Secondary prophylaxis

The actions of aspirin depend on the dose given. This varies between 75 mg/day and >3 g/day. Lower doses still can be tried for people who are normally intolerant of aspirin.

1. Anti-thrombotic effects are achieved by low dose treatment, i.e. 160–325 mg/day, by inhibition of thromboxane A.
2. Analgesic effects are achieved by moderate doses, i.e. 1–3 g/day.
3. Non-steroidal anti-inflammatory effects are achieved at high doses, i.e. 3 or more g/day, but aspirin becomes pro-thrombotic at these levels (by diminishing prostacyclin formation).

The adverse effects associated with aspirin, i.e. gastrointestinal bleeding, and possible exacerbation of peptic ulcers, are rare and insignificant at low, anti-thrombotic doses.

4.2.5 Atropine

Indications for use:
Bradycardia with hypotension
Asystole (second drug in algorithm.)

The recommended adult dose for symptomatic bradycardia is 0.5–1 mg IV, and for asystole it is 3 mg IV. The endotracheal route may be used as an emergency and 2–3 times the IV dose should be given.

Atropine competes with the parasympathetic neurotransmitter, acetylcholine, to block muscarinic receptor sites. The cardiac effects of atropine are mediated by vagal inhibition at the level of the S-A and A-V nodes. Increases in heart rate and (rate related) cardiac output occur. The blood pressure may rise as a secondary phenomenon.

Other effects of atropine become more prominent as the dose increases. They are not relevant to the cardiac arrest situation. Note that dilated pupils in a post-arrest patient should not be attributed solely to the use of atropine. However, a successfully treated bradycardic patient may well complain of blurred vision or a dry mouth, or develop retention of urine.

Paediatric doses are 20 µg/kg (0.02 mg/kg) IV or 40 µg/kg if given endotracheally.

4.2.6 Beta-blockers

Indications for use:
Unstable angina
Second-line treatment for supraventricular tachycardia (SVT)

There are numerous types of beta-blocking drugs, with different proportions of β_1 to β_2 antagonist activity.

4.2.6.1 First generation agents

These first generation agents, such as propranolol, non-selectively block β_1 and β_2 receptors to reduce heart rate by antagonism of circulating catecholamines and by reducing the rate of conduction across the A-V node. They have a negative inotropic effect, i.e. reduce cardiac contractility. Antagonism of bronchiolar β_2 receptors may lead to significant bronchospasm in susceptible individuals. The half-life of propranolol is 3 h. The dose for treatment of an SVT is 1 mg IV, repeated once if necessary.

4.2.6.2 Second generation agents

These are relatively cardioselective, i.e. block β_1 receptors almost exclusively, although this benefit is lost at high doses. An example is atenolol and the usual dose is 50–100 mg/day, orally.

4.2.6.3 Third generation agents

The third generation agents are relatively cardioselective, but also have some vasodilatory properties, mediated through partial agonist activity on β_2 receptors in arterial vessel walls.

The use of any beta-blocker may precipitate left ventricular failure in patients with an already failing ventricle, hypotension, or heart block. Profound bradycardia may develop at higher doses and be difficult to treat. The risk of heart block or asystole is increased if IV verapamil is used in a beta-blocked patient, especially if the beta-blocker dose was given intravenously.

Thus, care is required in treatment of SVT, a non-life-threatening condition, in order to avoid converting it into a life-threatening condition by injudicious poly-pharmacy.

The benefit of using beta-blockers after myocardial infarction (MI) to treat tachycardia with persistent hypertension and ventricular arrhythmias was clearly shown by the ISIS 1 study.

4.2.7 Bretylium tosylate

Indications for use:
Refractory ventricular tachycardia (VT) and ventricular fibrillation (VF)

Bretylium tosylate is a class III anti-arrhythmic agent which acts mainly on Purkinje fibres and less on ventricular muscle. It is taken up by terminal sympathetic neurons and initially causes the release of stored noradrenaline. This may transiently cause a deterioration in the rhythm. It is then stored in the nerve terminals and, because it prevents further neurotransmitter release, is said to cause a 'chemical sympathectomy'.

It may take 30 min to achieve its effect and so use of this drug in a cardiac arrest commits the resuscitation team to continuing their efforts for 30 min at least from the time of injection. The initial dose is 5 mg/kg. If successful, this should be followed by an infusion of 1–2 mg/kg/h. The half-life is 7–9 h. The major troublesome side effects are postural hypotension and nausea.

4.2.8 Calcium

Indications for use:
In electromechanical dissociation, use after adrenaline if due to:

severe hyperkalaemia
severe hypocalcaemia
overdose of Ca^{2+} channel blockers

At present doses of 10 ml 10% calcium chloride by minijet (6.8 mmol Ca^{2+}) or 20–30 ml calcium gluconate are recommended.

Calcium assists in coupling and uncoupling of muscle fibrils during contractions. *In vitro*, calcium will both restart an arrested heart preparation and cause marked cerebral and coronary arterial vasospasm. Calcium is therefore given during cardiac resuscitation only when a specific indication is present or strongly suspected.

The reason for the difference in given doses is that calcium chloride solutions contain approximately twice the concentration of calcium compared with gluconate solutions.

Calcium chloride should not be given immediately before or after sodium bicarbonate, without first flushing the line. This prevents precipitation within the IV line or cannula.

Note that digoxin toxicity is aggravated by a high serum calcium.

4.2.9 Diazepam

Indications for use:
To stop convulsions

Diazepam is a benzodiazepine agent which has some modest sedative and good anticonvulsant activity.

10–20 mg should be given IV at 1 mg/min. In children, if IV access is difficult it can be given rectally. The paediatric doses are 0.25 mg/kg at 1 mg/min IV or twice that for rectal administration. These doses can be repeated once if necessary.

Diazepam has no place in the post-arrest period unless the patient is fitting.

4.2.10 Digoxin

Indications for use:
Atrial fibrillation with fast ventricular response
Chronic left ventricular failure

Digoxin is a cardiac glycoside which enhances myocardial contractility and slows the ventricular rate by slowing both the sino-atrial discharge rate and the rate of conduction across the A-V node.

Rapid digitalization can be achieved by a combination of IV and oral loading doses. A dose of 0.5 mg digoxin in 50 ml 5% dextrose is given IV over 1 h, followed by 0.25 mg orally once or twice until 0.75 mg or 1.0 mg has been given in 24 h. If the patient is small, old, frail or has any renal impairment, a lower dose must be used. Oral maintenance doses usually lie between 0.0625 mg and 0.5 mg per day. The half-life of digoxin is 36 h.

Side effects increase in severity as the serum levels rise. They include nausea, anorexia, confusion, dizziness and arrhythmias. A wide variety of arrhythmias may develop, from paroxysmal atrial tachycardia with varying degrees of block to ventricular ectopics and bigemini. Digoxin toxicity can be confirmed by direct measurement of blood levels. Toxicity is increased by hypokalaemia, hypomagnesaemia, hypoxia, renal failure or hypercalcaemia.

See Chapter 10 for the treatment of digoxin toxicity.

4.2.11 Frusemide

Indications for use:
Left ventricular failure (LVF)
Congestive heart failure
To produce a diuresis

Frusemide is a diuretic which acts on the ascending limb of the loop of Henle to produce a diuresis within 10–20 min of an intravenous injection. It is more powerful than thiazide diuretics, and can produce a response even when the glomerular filtration rate is low. Another important action is venodilatation with a consequent reduction in myocardial preload. This precedes the diuretic action and is why a patient with acute pulmonary oedema/LVF feels less breathless even before the urine output has increased.

The adult dose required varies from 20 mg to 120 mg IV. In children, the dose is 1 mg/kg.

As long as hypovolaemia has been excluded, anuria is not a contraindication to the use of frusemide. Hypokalaemia may develop during treatment and precipitate arrhythmias, especially when used early after MI, or if the patient is already digitalized. Therefore, careful attention must be given to IV or oral potassium replacement, noting that the normal daily requirements for an adult are between 40 and 80 mmol of potassium per day.

4.2.12 Inotropic agents

Rational use of both inotropic agents requires the use of invasive monitoring since their actions may be unpredictable.

4.2.12.1 Dopamine

Indications for use:
Hypotension not due to simple hypovolaemia
To promote a diuresis

Dopamine is a positive inotrope which has an agonist effect on dopamine, α and β_1 receptors of the sympathetic nervous system. Alpha effects may predominate at higher doses. Low doses may increase renal blood flow due to inotropic (β_1) effects, but the diuretic action is probably not purely a result of this, but due more to stimulation of dopamine receptors in the renal tubules.

The usual starting dose is 2 μg/kg/min, and increased as necessary to achieve the desired effect.

The 'renal' dose range is 1–3 μg/kg/min; the inotropic dose is 3–10 μg/kg/min and α agonist effects predominate over 10 μg/kg/min.

The paediatric dose is 2–10 μg/kg (up to 0.01 mg/kg).

Dopamine has the potential to increase myocardial oxygen demand beyond the supply. Thus dopamine can be arrhythmogenic and may even increase the size of an infarct. It tends to increase cardiac filling pressures, which is a disadvantage in a failing heart.

4.2.12.2 Dobutamine

Indications for use:
Hypotension not due to simple hypovolaemia
Cardiogenic shock

Dobutamine is a positive inotrope affecting mainly β_1 receptors. Its advantage when compared with dopamine is that it tends to lower cardiac filling pressures and usually the peripheral vascular resistance is reduced. However, there is the same potential as with dopamine for increasing myocardial oxygen demand beyond supply, for increasing infarct size, and inducing arrhythmias. The dose starts at 2.5 μg/kg/min and is increased gradually, until the desired effect is achieved.

4.2.13 Isoprenaline

Indications for use:
Symptomatic bradycardia, unresponsive to atropine

Isoprenaline is a pure β_1 and β_2 agonist, with no α activity. It is more chronotropic than inotropic (β_1 effects) and also reduces peripheral vascular resistance by dilating vessels in the splanchnic circulation and skeletal muscle (β_2 effects). It is not a first-line drug. It is used only when atropine has failed, and some improvement in the patient's condition is required in the interim before internal pacing is carried out.

If 2 mg isoprenaline is mixed in 500 ml 5% dextrose, this yields a 4 μg/ml solution. This is infused at 2–10 μg/min, (i.e. 0.5–2.5 ml/min). The half-life is approximately 2 min.

The disadvantages of isoprenaline are: bradycardia may be converted to a fast tachycardia, giving little time for coronary artery filling; myocardial excitability is increased, resulting in a tendency to develop arrhythmias; and there is a redistribution of blood volume away from vital organs.

4.2.14 Lignocaine

Indications for use:
Haemodynamically stable ventricular tachycardia (VT), first-line
Refractory ventricular fibrillation (VF)

An initial bolus dose of 100 mg is given to an adult. This is repeated once and followed, if necessary, by an infusion of 2–4 mg/min.

Lignocaine is a class IB anti-arrhythmic agent, because it inhibits the fast sodium current and shortens the duration of the action potential. It acts selectively in diseased and ischaemic tissue, interrupting and preventing re-entry circuits. Lignocaine acts to stabilize cell membranes and is a good local anaesthetic.

Lignocaine is metabolized very rapidly by the liver, which makes the oral route of administration useless. For arrhythmia management, it must be given intravenously. An initial bolus of 100 mg is rapidly distributed throughout the body, and is effective for approximately 10 min. It must be followed by a second bolus of 100 mg, and then an infusion of 2–4 mg/min. The half-life is then 2 h, unless liver blood flow is reduced. Then the duration of action is prolonged. The paediatric dose is 1 mg/kg. Lignocaine is less effective in the presence of hypokalaemia and hypomagnesaemia.

At higher rates of infusion, the patient may feel dizzy, notice difficulty in speaking, numbness around the mouth or become drowsy. If blood levels rise further, convulsions occur and death ensues. Such side effects are more common in patients over the age of 60 years. Even when using lignocaine as a local anaesthetic it is worth remembering that the maximum safe dose in a normal person is 3 mg/kg.

4.2.15 Naloxone

Indications for use:
Opiate overdose

Naloxone is a specific opiate antagonist, which is extremely effective. Its duration of action is very short in comparison with the drugs whose effects it reverses, so that an initial IV dose must be followed by subcutaneous, IM or further IV boluses or an infusion.

Children require a dose of 0.01–0.04 mg/kg given IV. For adults, use 0.8–2 mg IV initially, and repeated every 2–3 min if necessary, to a maximum of 10 mg. Alternatively, an infusion can be used, adjusting the rate to achieve the desired effect.

4.2.16 Nitrates

Indications for use:
Unstable angina
Acute myocardial infarction, for analgesia
Left ventricular failure (LVF)

Nitrates act on vascular smooth muscle to cause relaxation. This dilatation is more marked on the venous than the arterial side of the circulation, so that myocardial preload is reduced proportionately more than afterload. Nitrates also dilate the coronary arteries, relieving spasm and redistributing flow from epicardial to endocardial regions by opening up collateral channels.

There are several routes of administration for nitrates: transdermal, buccal and sublingual, oral and intravenous infusion. Nitrates delivered via buccal and sublingual routes are useful in the acute situation, beginning to be effective within 1–2 min. The duration of action depends on the nitrate used and mode of delivery. Side effects include flushing, headaches and, sometimes, hypotension. Nitrates should not be used in patients who are already hypotensive. Examples of nitroglycerine doses are given:

Buccal tablets 3–5 mg. (Remove if the blood pressure drops)
IV infusion (Tridil) 0.3–12 mg/h. (Stop or slow infusion if blood pressure drops)

Sublingual GTN spray 0.4 mg metered dose used twice is very effective but has the disadvantage that the dose cannot be adjusted if the patient becomes hypotensive.

4.2.17 Opiates

Indications for use:
Analgesia
Acute left ventricular failure (LVF)

Morphine and diamorphine are both opiate analgesics. Morphine has a vasodilator activity which reduces preload and therefore myocardial oxygen demand. However, in the presence of hypovolaemia, it may cause profound hypotension. Adult doses of 2.5–10 mg diamorphine are equipotent to 5–20 mg morphine. Paediatric doses should be based on 100 µg/kg (= 0.1 mg/kg) for morphine and 50 µg/kg (= 0.05 mg/kg) for diamorphine.

Opiates should be given by slow IV injection with the actual dose being titrated against the degree of pain relief achieved. This should prevent the sudden onset of profound respiratory depression, hypotension or bradycardia. The size of the dose will also depend on the age and size of the patient.

Respiratory depression or hypotension can be reversed by subcutaneous, IM or IV naloxone 0.8 mg (2 × 0.4 mg ampoules).

4.2.18 Phenytoin

Indications for use:
Digoxin-induced arrhythmias
Third-line drug in paediatrics for convulsions

Phenytoin is an anticonvulsant agent which also has some class IB anti-arrhythmic activity. However, if injected too quickly, it can also cause arrhythmias. It is particularly useful in treating ventricular dysrhythmias occurring as a result of digoxin toxicity, and after congenital heart surgery in children.

It is a third-line drug for the treatment of convulsions in paediatrics.

In both adults and children, the loading dose is 10–15 mg/kg, diluted in normal saline and given over 20–30 min. The patient should be attached to a cardiac monitor to assess their response to treatment. Maintenance doses are 400–600 mg daily for adults and 5 mg/kg/day for children. The peak effect occurs early, at 15–20 min after injection, but it has a long half-life, allowing a once daily dose.

Phenytoin induces hepatic enzymes and may alter the dose requirements of some drugs, e.g. lignocaine.

4.2.19 Sodium bicarbonate

Indications for use:
Severe metabolic acidosis

In adults, if the pH is <7.0–7.1 during or immediately following resuscitation for cardiac arrest, small doses of sodium bicarbonate are sometimes given. The dose required in mmol sodium bicarbonate 8.4% solution is:

$$\frac{\text{base excess} \times \text{weight (kg)}}{3} \tag{4.1}$$

Smaller doses of 50 mmol (50 ml 8.4% $NaHCO_3$) are given and repeated as required guided by regular blood gas monitoring. The paediatric dose is 1 mmol/kg (1 ml of 8.4% solution/kg).

A value of 8.4% sodium bicarbonate presents a high and osmotically active sodium level to an already compromised circulation and brain. Because a mild acidosis causes cerebral vasodilatation and possibly an increased cerebral blood flow, full correction of the pH could potentially result in diminution of the cerebral blood flow at a particularly critical time. The bicarbonate ion is excreted as CO_2 via the lungs, so that ventilation must be increased correspondingly. Intracellular acidosis is increased by bicarbonate administration. Thus a metabolic acidosis must be severe to warrant giving sodium bicarbonate.

4.2.20 Thrombolytic therapy

Indications for use:
Myocardial salvage

1. Streptokinase
2. Alteplase (tPA)
3. Anistreplase (acetylated streptokinase)

Thrombolytic therapy is the only available treatment that directly influences the outcome of MI by reducing the size of the infarct. The sooner it is used from the onset of chest pain (0–6 h), the better the results, although some benefit is still obtained up to 24 h later. The therapy is still more effective when used in combination with aspirin, 160 mg daily. Thus it should be given to everyone with strong evidence of MI, if none of the five specific contraindications are present.

4.2.20.1 Contraindications

1. The patient has had a recent haemorrhage or has a bleeding disorder.
2. The patient has undergone recent invasive procedures.
3. The patient is comatosed and intracranial haemorrhage cannot be excluded as the cause.
4. There is potential for emboli to be thrown off as intramural thrombus is thrombolysed.
5. The patient has profound hypotension (for streptokinase and anistreplase but not for tPA).

A recent streptococcal infection is a relative contraindication.

Possible consequences of the use of thrombolytic agents are bleeding or allergy. Streptokinase and anistreplase are the two agents most likely to provoke an allergic reaction, and so they are always used together with IV hydrocortisone and antihistamines. Reperfusion arrhythmias are common with each agent, when successful.

Streptokinase is the cheapest and has been shown to be as effective as the other agents. It is therefore the agent of choice.

However, tPA is non-antigenic, does not cause hypotension, and does not require an infusion, and this becomes the agent of choice if the patient has had a streptokinase infusion in the previous 12 months or a more recent streptococcal infection.

4.2.21 Verapamil

Indications for use:
Supraventricular tachycardia (SVT)
Angina

The dose is 5–15 mg when given intravenously. It should be diluted to 1 mg/ml with saline and given slowly, to a monitored patient.

Verapamil is a class IV anti-arrhythmic agent. It is a calcium channel blocking drug and therefore a coronary artery and peripheral vasodilator. It reduces conduction through the A-V node. Verapamil has a significant negative inotropic effect, which is the reason why it should not be given to a patient with a broad complex tachycardia of ventricular origin.

Side effects are those of any vasodilators, i.e. flushing, headaches and hypotension.

The hypotensive effects last for only 5–10 min, but they can be dramatic: anti-arrhythmic effects persist for about 6 h after an IV bolus.

Drug interactions with digoxin and beta-blockers are most pronounced in association with IV verapamil.

Verapamil interacts with digoxin, causing digoxin plasma levels to rise. Both drugs have an additive effect on the A-V node. If digoxin levels are high, this can lead to asystole.

Although verapamil and beta-blockers are successfully used together orally to treat hypertension and angina, if given IV there is an additive negative inotropic effect with resultant severe, refractory hypotension. This may also develop if verapamil is used in combination with any other anti-arrhythmic agent which also has a negative inotropic effect.

4.3 PAEDIATRIC DOSES

Adrenaline: 10–100 µg/kg IV or via intraosseous route.

Adenosine: 25 µg/kg as an IV bolus, followed every 2 min by 50 µg/kg increments until success has been achieved or a maximum dose of 500 µg/kg has been given.

Amiodarone: 5 mg/kg over 30 min IV, followed by 625 µg/kg/h.

Atropine: 20 µg/kg IV or via intraosseous route.

Bretylium: 5 mg/kg IV bolus followed by 1–2 mg/kg/h.

Beta-blockers:

Propranolol: 10–50 µg/kg very slowly IV, for tachy-arrhythmias if pacing is not available. Do not mix with verapamil.

Calcium:

If 10% calcium chloride solution is used, the dose is 0.1 ml/kg (0.68 mmol/ml).

If 10% calcium gluconate solution is used, the dose is 0.2 ml/kg (0.225 mmol/ml).

Diazepam: 0.25 mg/kg IV at 1 mg/min or 0.5 mg/kg rectally.

Digoxin: Use 10 µg/kg in three divided doses in the first 24 h, to digitalize a child. This should be followed by a maintenance dose of 4 µg/kg (maximum dose 250 µg).

Dopamine/Dobutamine: 1–20 µg/kg/min.

Frusemide: 1 mg/kg IV.

Isoprenaline: 0.05–0.5 µg/kg/min IV.

Lignocaine: 1 mg/kg IV.

Opiates:

Diamorphine: 0.05 mg/kg.
Morphine: 0.1 mg/kg.

Naloxone: 0.01–0.04 mg/kg.

Phenytoin: 15 mg/kg IV diluted in saline, over 20–30 min (use continuous cardiac monitoring).

Sodium bicarbonate: 1 mmol/kg.

Verapamil: The normally increased sensitivity of a child's S-A and A-V nodes mean that there is a small but significant risk of inducing asystole by using verapamil. Consequently it is safer to keep verapamil as second- or third-line treatment for SVT in children.

5

Acid–base balance and arterial blood gas analysis

Objectives

After studying this chapter you should be able to:

- Understand the basic theory of acid–base balance

- Understand the reasons for acidosis following a cardiac arrest

- Understand the possible errors in sampling an arterial blood gas specimen

- Understand the interpretation of blood gas results

- Understand the management of the acid–base imbalance during and after cardiopulmonary resuscitation

- Demonstrate the ability to interpret acid–base data

In a cardiac arrest the main acid–base abnormality is acute acidosis. Therefore this chapter will concentrate on this aspect. The interested reader should look at Appendix C for a more comprehensive view of acidosis and alkalosis.

5.1 BASIC THEORY OF ACID–BASE BALANCE

The first step in understanding this subject is to comprehend certain key words and phrases.

5.1.1 Acids and bases

Originally the word 'acid' was used to describe the sour taste of unripe fruit, but subsequently many different meanings were attributed to it. This led to considerable confusion and misunderstanding, which was not resolved until 1923, when the following definitions were proposed:

An acid is a substance which is capable of providing hydrogen ions (H^+).

A base is a substance which is capable of accepting hydrogen ions.

A strong acid, therefore, is a chemical which will readily provide many H^+ ions. Conversely, a strong base is a chemical which will readily accept many H^+ ions.

The concentration of hydrogen ions in solution is expressed with the symbol $[H^+]$.

5.1.2 The pH scale

The concentration of hydrogen ions in solution is usually very small, even with strong acids. Therefore, when one considers the weaker acids found in the body, H^+ concentrations in the order of 0.000 000 04 moles per litre are found. Dealing with these unwieldy numbers is obviously difficult, and so in 1909 the pH scale was developed. This scale had the advantage of being able to express any $[H^+]$ as a number between 0 and 14 (inclusive). This was achieved by representing the inverse H^+ concentration as its logarithmic value (see appendix C).

The normal range of arterial pH is 7.36–7.44, with an increase above 7.44 known as an alkalosis and a decrease below 7.36 known as an acidosis.

As the [H+] increases, the pH decreases.
Since pH is a logarithmic scale, small changes represent large changes in [H+].

5.1.3 Normal acid production

In human physiology, CO_2 produced during oxidative metabolism combines with water to produce carbonic acid, which then dissociates to hydrogen and bicarbonate ions. This can be expressed by the following equation:

$$H_2O + CO_2 \rightleftharpoons H_2CO_3 \rightleftharpoons H^+ + HCO_3^- \tag{5.1}$$

The combination of CO_2 with water is catalysed by the enzyme carbonic anhydrase. This is found in high concentrations in red blood cells, where it facilitates the rapid transfer of CO_2 between tissues, blood and alveolar gas.

The normal ratio of bicarbonate to carbonic acid is 20:1. In order for this ratio to be maintained, CO_2 must be delivered to the lungs where it can be removed by ventilation. Therefore, defects in ventilation or poor pulmonary perfusion will reduce the body's ability to eliminate hydrogen ions.

5.2 THE BODY'S RESPONSE TO AN ACID

Life is based on a series of complex chemical reactions controlled by special proteins called enzymes. The activity of an enzyme is affected by the acidity of its environment such that extreme acid or base abnormalities can lead to reduced metabolic activity and ultimately death.

The pH of the blood must therefore be kept within a very narrow band (7.36–7.44), even though potentially vast quantities of hydrogen ions are produced each day by normal metabolic activity. This control is achieved by a series of interlinked processes involving buffers, the lungs and the kidneys.

The first acute compensatory mechanism following an acid or alkali insult is the buffering system.

The second acute compensatory mechanism ameliorates pH changes by respiratory alterations.

Chronic compensation occurs, if the initial source of the acid–base imbalance persists, by the actions of the renal system.

It is important to realize that these measures never over-compensate. An acidosis remains an acidosis and an alkalosis always remains an alkalosis.

5.2.1 Buffers

These provide the body with a temporary, but very effective way of minimizing fluctuations in acidity. They work by taking up the free H^+ ions and transporting them to their place of elimination.

Intracellularly, the main buffers are proteins, phosphate and haemoglobin, but extracellularly the most important one is carbonic acid:

$$H_2O + CO_2 \rightleftharpoons H_2CO_3 \rightleftharpoons H^+ + HCO_3^- \qquad (5.2)$$

As mentioned previously, the ratio of HCO_3^- to H_2CO_3 is 20:1.

This means there is a large reserve of base available to neutralize the addition of any acid. However, in the ventilated patient, this reserve will be quickly used up if the kidneys cannot excrete the excess H^+ and regenerate the bicarbonate within a few hours.

The carbonic acid–bicarbonate buffer system has two important features:

1. Bicarbonate is present in great quantities in the body and it is therefore particularly important for rapid, fine-tuning adjustments of the extracellular pH.
2. Carbonic acid produces CO_2 which can be excreted by the lungs. Therefore the equivalent of a large acid load can be removed, provided the respiratory system is functioning normally.

5.2.2 Lungs

The potential respiratory acid load in a normal person amounts to 12 000 mmol/day. With 83 mmol H^+ being produced each hour, it is easy to see why there is a rapid onset of acidosis during episodes of hypoventilation.

The respiratory centre is extremely sensitive to a fall in pH or an increase in the arterial partial pressure of carbon dioxide ($PaCO_2$). Stimulation of the centre leads to a rapid increase in the rate and depth of ventilation.

5.2.3 Kidneys

The H^+ produced from other normal metabolic acid sources, such as lactate, fixed acids and urea synthesis, is approximately 3000 mmol/day. This acid load is excreted via the kidneys.

The renal tubular cells both secrete hydrogen ions into the glomerular filtrate and regenerate bicarbonate. However this takes much longer than the lungs to work (24–36 hours as opposed to minutes). In a chronic situation, it will take several days for the kidneys to adapt fully to the acid–base imbalance.

5.3 TYPES OF ACIDOSIS

5.3.1 Metabolic acidosis

This usually results from the accumulation of metabolic acids, for example, lactic acid following a cardiac arrest. This leads to a reduction in the serum bicarbonate, a rise in the carbonic acid and ultimately a rise in the $PaCO_2$:

$$\uparrow H^+ + HCO_3^- \rightleftharpoons \uparrow H_2CO_3 \rightleftharpoons \uparrow H_2O + \uparrow CO_2 \qquad (5.3)$$

As noted above, the rise in $PaCO_2$ leads to an increase in the minute ventilation with a subsequent reduction in the $PaCO_2$ within minutes.

The latter is known as **compensatory respiratory alkalosis** and it helps restore the pH to normal. Remember, though, the body never over-compensates, therefore the plasma pH will still be slightly acidic (less than 7.35). Even after several hours, respiratory compensation may be only 75% complete. Factors limiting the degree of respiratory compensation are the work involved in breathing and the systemic effects of hypocarbia.

An example of respiratory compensation is the deep respiratory excursions (Kussmaul's breathing) seen in ketoacidosis.

In the ensuing hours and days the kidneys will excrete the excess hydrogen ions and regenerate bicarbonate so that a near normal pH is restored.

Metabolic acidosis produces a fall in arterial pH and bicarbonate concentration. The compensatory respiratory alkalosis which subsequently occurs produces a decrease in the $PaCO_2$.

5.3.2 Respiratory acidosis

This occurs when there is a mismatch between carbon dioxide production and alveolar ventilation. An example of this is a cardiorespiratory arrest. It leads to a rise in the $PaCO_2$ and an increase in the hydrogen ion concentration as the following equation is forced to the right:

$$H_2O + CO_2 \rightleftharpoons H_2CO_3 \rightleftharpoons H^+ + HCO_3^- \qquad (5.4)$$

In the acute phase there is very little change in the plasma bicarbonate concentration. However, with time, the kidneys can compensate by increasing the absorption of bicarbonate. This is known as **compensatory metabolic alkalosis** and it leads to a rise in the plasma bicarbonate concentration. Remember the body never over-compensates, therefore the arterial pH is still slightly acidic.

It is important to realize that the carbonic acid buffer system does not buffer respiratory acid production – an acid cannot react with its own salt. Instead other buffers are used.

Respiratory acidosis leads to a fall in the arterial pH and a rise in the $PaCO_2$. There is eventually also a metabolic compensatory alkalosis which produces a rise in the plasma bicarbonate concentration.

5.3.3 Combined respiratory and metabolic acidosis

Following a cardiac arrest, acidosis results from both a respiratory and a metabolic cause. These can add together to produce disturbances in the patient's acid–base balance which lie outside the compensatory limits occurring after a single cause.

To determine the metabolic component, the **base excess** (BE) is calculated. This is defined as the number of moles of acid or alkali which must be added to 1 litre of blood so that a pH of 7.4 is produced. Respiratory influences are eliminated by keeping the $PaCO_2$ constant at 40 mmHg (5.3 kPa). The BE should be zero but, in metabolic acidosis, bicarbonate needs to be added to the blood to restore the pH. This amount is expressed as a negative value and is called a **base deficit**. Conversely, in metabolic alkalosis, acid needs to be added and so the amount is expressed as a positive value.

The base deficit is used to help calculate the dose of bicarbonate which should be given to a patient to correct the metabolic acidosis.

5.3.4 Metabolic alkalosis

This follows either a loss of metabolic acids (e.g. vomiting), or a gain in bicarbonate (e.g. excessive administration of sodium bicarbonate).

In an attempt to try and correct the alkalosis, there is a **compensatory respiratory acidosis.** This results in hypoventilation and a rise in the $PaCO_2$. Respiratory compensation is limited by the hypoxaemia which results from the hypoventilation.

Long-term compensation is by excretion of excess bicarbonate by the kidneys.

Metabolic alkalosis produces a direct rise in arterial pH and bicarbonate. Later a compensatory respiratory acidosis occurs producing an increase in the $PaCO_2$.

5.4 PRECAUTIONS WHEN TAKING AN ARTERIAL BLOOD GAS SAMPLE

The arterial blood gas (ABG) sample is essential for the accurate diagnosis of an acid–base disorder. It is therefore very important that the sample is taken and analysed correctly. Several iatrogenic errors need to be avoided:

1. **Ensure an adequate sample**. Samples taken from catheters should have any dead space discarded first. A 4 ml discard is sufficient for samples taken from arterial and central venous lines, and 6 ml for samples taken from a pulmonary artery catheter. A sample volume of 2 ml is adequate.
2. **Avoid excess heparin**. The use of too much heparin can lead to marked changes in the ABG analysis. It is adequate to fill the dead space of a 2 ml or 5 ml syringe, with needle attached, with 1:1000 heparin. The use of preheparinized syringes is recommended.
3. **Avoid contamination with room air**. Remove froth and large bubbles and then seal the syringe with a plastic cap. Allowing oxygen and carbon dioxide to diffuse in or out of the blood sample can alter the level in the blood within minutes.
4. **Minimize the effects of metabolism in the sample**. Any delay in the sample will allow oxygen to be consumed and carbon dioxide to be generated in the syringe. If a delay to analysis of more than 10 min is expected, the sample should be stored on ice.
5. **Obtain all available information**. It is not possible to sensibly interpret the PaO_2 unless the inspired oxygen fraction (FIO_2) is known. Any recent bicarbonate therapy should also be noted. Extremes of temperature can affect interpretation of ABG analysis since samples are analysed at 37°C and the relationship between content and partial pressure will change as the sample temperature changes.
6. **Avoid errors in analysis**. It is important to use machines which have been calibrated daily and subjected to regular quality control checks.

5.5 ANALYSIS OF THE ARTERIAL BLOOD GAS SAMPLE

The proper interpretation of a blood gas analysis requires a clinical history, examination and a review of the rest of the laboratory investigations. In the emergency situation much of this data will be lacking and one must interpret the initial results with caution and follow trends while other information is being obtained (Figure 5.1).

Fig. 5.1
Algorithm for
diagnosis of
common acid–base
disturbances
(mixed pictures
are not
uncommon)

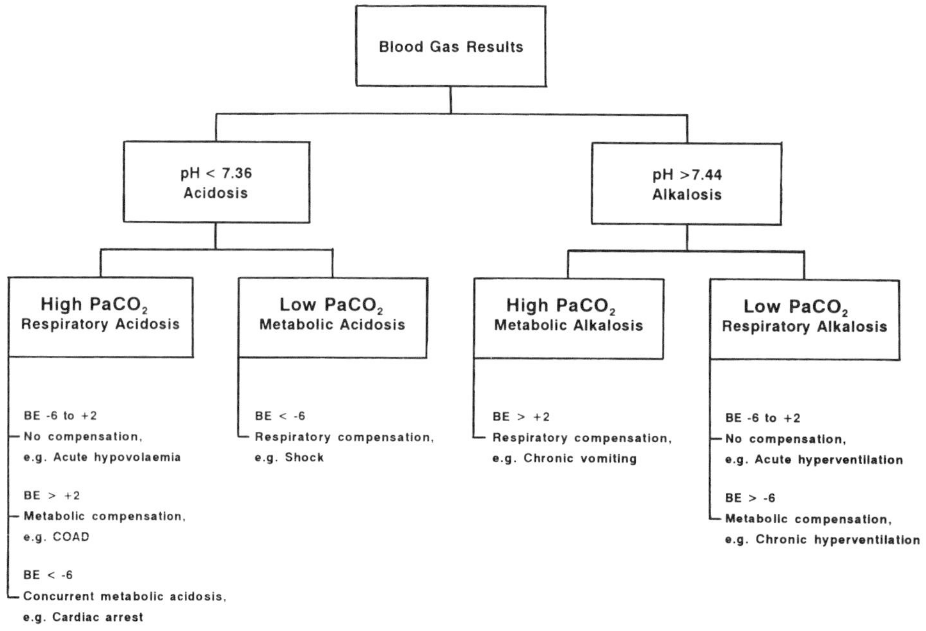

5.5.1 Check the pH (normal 7.36–7.44)

Is there an acidosis or alkalosis? If the pH is near normal it could be due to respiratory or metabolic compensation, but remember this is never complete.

5.5.2 Check the PaCO$_2$ (normal 35–45 mmHg or 4.7–6.0 kPa)

This gives a good indication of ventilatory adequacy because it is inversely proportional to alveolar minute volume (respiratory rate × alveolar tidal volume). When combined with the pH, it can be used to determine if there are primary or compensatory ventilatory changes.

5.5.3 Check the base excess (normal 0 ± 2 mmol)

Empirically a positive BE indicates a metabolic alkalosis and a negative BE (base deficit) a metabolic acidosis. However, a slight acidosis is beneficial because it facilitates the release of oxygen, from the haemoglobin molecule, to the tissues. Therefore a base deficit is only treated if it is large, i.e. more negative than −10.

Blood gas analysers utilize the Henderson equation to calculate bicarbonate and BE. Major therapeutic decisions based on these calculated values are unwise since there are inherent problems in extrapolating these experimental values to the real-life situation.

5.5.4 Check the PaO_2 (normal >80 mmHg or 10.6 kPa on air)

The partial pressure of oxygen in the arterial sample (PaO_2) is then interpreted in the light of the FIO_2. Since atmospheric pressure is approximately 100 kPa, 1% is about 1 kPa. This would mean that inspiring say 30% O_2 from a face-mask would lead to an alveolar concentration of approximately 20–25 kPa. (This apparent fall is because there is a normal drop of about 7.5 kPa between the oxygen partial pressure inspired at the mouth and that of the alveoli.) Anything significantly greater than about 5–10 kPa difference would imply there is a ventilation-perfusion mismatch in the lungs.

5.5.5 Examples

5.5.5.1

A 17-year-old schoolgirl is found at home by her parents in a restless and confused state. She is pale, sweaty and hyperventilating. Electrolytes and arterial blood gases while breathing room air are:

pH   7.10
$PaCO_2$ 2.4 kPa (18 mmHg)
PaO_2 14 kPa (105 mmHg)
BE   −14
Na   135
K   5.0
HCO_3 10
C   95

Interpretation:

What is the pH?   There is an acidosis.
What is the $PaCO_2$?   There is hypocarbia, i.e. this is not a respiratory acidosis and represents respiratory compensation.
What is the PaO_2?   The degree of oxygenation is normal.
What are the other data?   The anion gap is 35 (see Appendix C). The most likely cause of an increased anion gap acidosis in a previously healthy adolescent is an overdose (check the salicylate level) or diabetic ketoacidosis (check the blood sugar level).

5.5.5.2

A 19-year-old secretary with a history of asthma presents herself to the Accident and Emergency Department in a distressed state with severe dyspnoea. Arterial blood gases during oxygen therapy via a 28% Venturi mask are:

pH   7.5
$PaCO_2$ 2.4 kPa (18 mmHg)
PaO_2 22 kPa (165 mmHg)
BE   −3

Interpretation:

What is the pH? There is an alkalosis.
What is the $PaCO_2$? There is hypocarbia, i.e. there is a respiratory alkalosis.
What is the BE? The base excess is normal, i.e. this is not compensatory hyperventilation from a metabolic acidosis.
What is the PaO_2? The degree of oxygenation is normal. Asthma produces a reduced PaO_2.

The diagnosis is hysterical overbreathing.

5.6 MANAGEMENT OF ACID–BASE DISTURBANCES IN A CARDIAC ARREST

5.6.1 Types

There are three disturbances of acid–base balance that can occur during the treatment of a cardiac arrest:

1. Within minutes of a cardiac arrest, a respiratory acidosis occurs as a result of hypoventilation and a decrease in pulmonary blood flow. This leads to a reduction in CO_2 excretion and a fall in the end tidal CO_2 level. Consequently, carbon dioxide accumulates in the venous circulation and the central venous to arterial CO_2 gradient widens. Even with CPR, respiratory acidosis occurs because the cardiac output is rarely greater than 30% of normal.
2. Later a metabolic acidosis also supervenes because of the production of lactic acidosis.
3. Following endotracheal intubation and artificial ventilation, the reduced volume of CO_2 delivered to the alveoli, as described above, is easily cleared. This may lead to a condition known as **paradoxical respiratory alkalosis**. In this there is arterial hypocarbia despite the persistent venous acidosis due to the high venous concentration of CO_2 and lactic acid. The pH of the arterial blood can be neutral, mildly acidotic or even alkalotic. Indeed, severe arterial acidosis in a patient receiving CPR indicates there is inadequate ventilation/oxygenation of the patient.

It follows from this that a central venous gas sample should be used to determine the patient's pH following a cardiac arrest. The arterial blood gas sample should be used to assess the patient's oxygenation.

5.6.2 Initial treatment of acidosis

The respiratory and metabolic acidosis which results from a cardiac arrest should be treated initially with hyperventilation with 100% oxygen.

Bicarbonate is not the treatment of choice. When this is given intravenously it reacts with the hydrogen ions and increases local CO_2 production. Carbon dioxide rapidly diffuses into cells, and intracellular acidosis is worsened. Hypernatraemia and hyperosmolar states are also common following bicarbonate administration. Furthermore the arterial alkalosis, produced by the injection of bicarbonate, leads to a left shift of the oxyhaemoglobin dissociation curve and a reduction in the oxygen delivery to the tissues. For each 0.1 rise in pH there is a drop of around 10% in the tissue oxygen availability.

Treat the initial acidosis following a cardiac arrest with effective CPR and hyperventilation, not bicarbonate.

5.6.3 Later treatment of acidosis

The disparity between the level of acidosis measured in a central venous sample and that in an arterial sample becomes even more marked when there is a prolonged resuscitation (>10 min) or following restoration of the cardiac output. In the latter case, considerable quantities of lactic acid are 'washed out' of the peripheral tissues by the restored blood supply and carried to the central veins.

In these cases small doses of bicarbonate may occasionally be used, but increased ventilation will be required to excrete the excess CO_2 generated. The amount of bicarbonate (in mmol/l) to be given is determined by:

1. The value of the base excess greater than −10 (i.e. the lowest part of the normal range).
2. The size of the extracellular fluid volume. This is approximately a third of the body weight. Bicarbonate needed = (BE > −10) × body weight/3.

As 1 mmol = 1 ml of 8.4% HCO_3, this value is also the number of ml of 8.4% solution required to restore the pH of the extracellular fluid to normal.

Usually smaller doses (50 mmol) are given and the effect monitored by repeat blood gas analysis.

Although acid–base interpretation with CPR is generally a straightforward respiratory and metabolic acidosis, pre-existing disturbances may have been present or may even have contributed to the cause for the resuscitation.

5.7 SUMMARY

In general, acidosis is the dominant acid–base abnormality in patients suffering from a cardiac arrest. This must be managed with effective cardiopulmonary resuscitation and adequate ventilation.

The body's compensatory mechanism to an acid–base imbalance is to produce an acid–base state diametrically opposite to the primary problem:

A respiratory acidosis is compensated by a metabolic alkalosis.
A metabolic acidosis is compensated by a respiratory alkalosis.
A metabolic alkalosis is compensated by a respiratory acidosis.

Practical skill station
Acid–base balance

AIMS

To reinforce practically the knowledge of acid–base balance gained in theoretical sessions.

To allow candidates to work through practical examples of blood gas analysis.

TEACHING TECHNIQUE

A group discussion format is used, in which candidates are asked to demonstrate their knowledge and understanding of the analysis and interpretation of blood gas results.

TESTING

Candidates are informally assessed during the skill station. Formal assessment is not carried out separately; questions are included in the Multiple Choice Paper on the final day.

6

Airway control and ventilation

Objectives

After studying this chapter you should be able to:

- Perform basic support of the airway and ventilation

- Understand advanced airway control

- Understand advanced control of ventilation

- Demonstrate the use of advanced techniques of airway control

6.1 BASIC AIRWAY AND VENTILATORY SUPPORT

Control of the airway and the establishment of ventilation are essential prerequisites for successful resuscitation.

6.1.1 Airway support

When faced with an unconscious patient (no response to verbal or gentle physical stimulation), the first task is to ensure a patent airway. Failure to perform this simple procedure is a frequent cause of avoidable death in the unconscious patient. The commonest cause of airway obstruction is the tongue. In the unconscious patient, the reduction in muscle tone allows the tongue to fall backwards, thereby obstructing the pharynx (Figure 6.1).

Vomit, blood and inhaled foreign bodies may also cause acute obstruction. Soft tissue infections and local tumours usually cause airway obstruction more gradually. Using the basic life support techniques of head tilt and chin lift or jaw thrust (see Figures 2.4 and 2.7), airway patency will be restored in the majority of patients. The success of these actions in providing an airway should be ascertained quickly, by looking for movement of the chest, listening for breath sounds and feeling for expired air. Movement of the chest wall alone is not satisfactory, as paradoxical movement will occur with respiratory effort and an

53

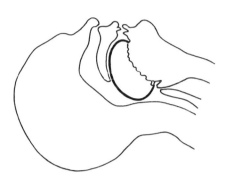

Fig. 6.1 Airway cross-section showing obstruction by the tongue

obstructed airway. If these actions fail to provide a clear airway, and breathing is noisy, a check must be made to ensure that obstruction is not due to foreign debris, and a finger sweep should be performed. If there is any evidence of trauma, the possible co-existence of a cervical injury must be remembered.

6.1.2 Airway adjuncts

Simple devices may be used to try to improve or help to maintain airway patency in patients who are breathing spontaneously or being ventilated. The commonest of these are the oropharyngeal (Guedel) and nasopharyngeal airways.

The oropharyngeal airway is made in a variety of sizes, those most commonly used being sizes 2, 3 and 4 for small to large adults. An estimate of the size required can be obtained by comparing the airway with the distance from the corner of the mouth to the angle of the jaw. The airway is usually inserted 'upside down' (concave uppermost) as far as the back of the hard palate. It is then rotated 180° and fully inserted until the flange lies in front of the upper and lower incisors (Figure 6.2).

Insertion may occasionally worsen airway obstruction, cause oral trauma and bleeding, or impact unrecognized foreign bodies further into the pharynx. In a patient who is not deeply unconscious an oropharyngeal airway may cause pharyngeal stimulation and vomiting.

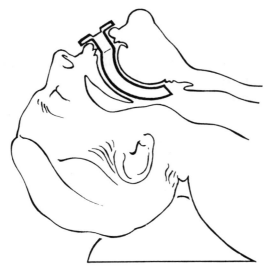

Fig. 6.2 Oral airway *in situ*

Nasopharyngeal airways are more malleable, and may be less stimulating. They are sized on their internal diameter in millimetres and the length increases with diameter. The range of sizes used in adults is generally from 6 mm to 8 mm (approximately the same diameter as the patient's little finger). Having lubricated the airway, it is inserted vertically along the floor of the nose, with a gentle twisting action, trying the right nostril first. Once in place, a safety pin can be inserted through the flanged end to prevent it being inhaled. Even with careful insertion, bleeding can be precipitated, usually from tissue in the nasopharynx. If the tube is too long, both vomiting and laryngospasm can be induced in patients who are not deeply unconscious (Figure 6.3).

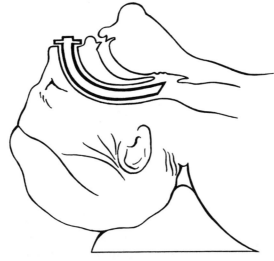

Fig. 6.3 Nasal airway *in situ*

A further problem of both these airways is that during assisted ventilation air can be directed down the oesophagus. This results in inefficient ventilation of the lungs, and gastric dilatation. In turn this splints the diaphragm, making ventilation difficult and may predispose to regurgitation of gastric contents. Consequently, immediately after inserting an oral or nasal airway, one should check to ensure that ventilation is being achieved (look, listen and feel), and that no complications have been caused.

55

6.1.3 Ventilatory support

When spontaneous ventilation commences following these manoeuvres, patients should be placed in an appropriate recovery position, where there will be less risk of further pharyngeal obstruction and vomit or blood will drain from the mouth.

6.1.3.1 Exhaled air resuscitation

If spontaneous ventilation is inadequate or absent, then artificial ventilation must be commenced. Expired air ventilation, which provides 16% oxygen, should be started immediately. This can be performed without any equipment using the mouth-to-mouth technique. A variety of devices are available which can be interposed between the rescuer and the patient to make expired air ventilation more acceptable, by reducing the risk of exposing the rescuer to vomit and infection. Higher concentrations of oxygen can be delivered when using a mouth-to-mask technique by attaching an oxygen supply to the mask (Figure 6.4).

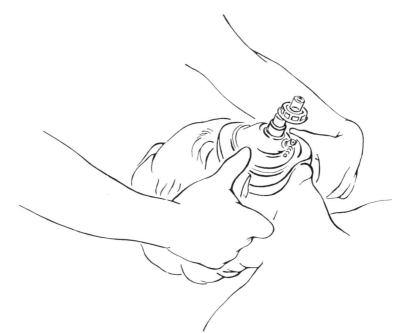

Fig. 6.4 Mouth-to-mask ventilation

6.1.3.2 Oxygen

Oxygen should be administered to all patients during resuscitation, with the aim being to increase inspired concentration to 100%. The concentration achieved will depend upon the system used and flow of oxygen available. For spontaneously breathing patients, a Venturi face-mask will deliver a fixed concentration (24% to 60%) depending on the mask chosen. Nasal cannulae can raise the oxygen concentration to 44% and a standard (concentration) mask will deliver up to 60%, providing the flow of oxygen is high enough (12–15 l/min). By using this type of mask with a non-rebreathing reservoir the inspired concentration can be raised to 85%, which makes it the most desirable method.

6.2 ADVANCED AIRWAY CONTROL AND VENTILATION

6.2.1 Airway control

In the deeply unconscious patient, the best way of controlling the airway is by tracheal intubation. This technique requires a greater degree of skill and more equipment than for the methods used in BLS. Tracheal intubation may be indicated for a variety of reasons. The most obvious is that other methods of providing an airway have failed. The airway may also need to be protected from the risk of aspiration of regurgitated stomach contents (during CPR), or from bleeding. Furthermore, the decision may be taken at an early stage in the resuscitation that there is the need for a period of prolonged ventilation (e.g. with certain types of poisoning). Occasionally tracheal intubation may prove impossible due to obstruction of the view of the larynx (e.g. abnormal anatomy, glottic oedema, laryngeal trauma or bleeding). In these circumstances, consideration must be given to the creation of a surgical airway, using either a large bore cannula or a knife to puncture the cricothyroid membrane (cricothyroidotomy).

6.2.1.1 Tracheal intubation

During CPR, tracheal intubation is the preferred method for controlling the airway. By isolating the airway, the risk of contamination is reduced, ventilation facilitated and gastric dilatation eliminated. In addition, the airway can be suctioned to remove secretions or inhaled debris and, in the patient in whom venous access is difficult, the tracheal tube provides an acceptable alternative route for the administration of some drugs (providing adjustment is made in the dosage). Tracheal intubation can be performed either orally or nasally. Oral intubation is generally the most common route during CPR. (In the multiply injured patient who is breathing spontaneously and in whom the possibility of a cervical fracture exists, consideration should be given to the nasal route.)

Whichever route is used, a variety of equipment is needed to facilitate intubation (see Annex A). It is essential that all equipment is checked on a regular basis and again prior to attempting intubation to ensure that everything required is at hand and functioning. Although a brief description of tracheal intubation via the oral route is included for completeness, this is not intended as a substitute for practice using a manikin or, better still, an anaesthetized patient under the direction of a skilled anaesthetist.

6.2.1.2 Technique

Whenever possible, intubation should be preceded by a period of ventilation with 100% oxygen, using a bag–valve–mask device. The patient is then positioned to facilitate intubation, with the neck flexed and the head extended at the atlanto-occipital joint ('sniffing the morning air'). Holding the laryngoscope in the left hand, the mouth should be opened and the blade of the laryngoscope introduced into the right-hand side of the mouth, displacing the tongue to the left. The blade is passed along the edge of the tongue and the tip of the epiglottis should be seen emerging at the base of the tongue. The blade is then advanced between the base of the tongue and the anterior surface of the epiglottis (vallecula). The tongue and epiglottis are then lifted to reveal the vocal cords (Figure 6.5).

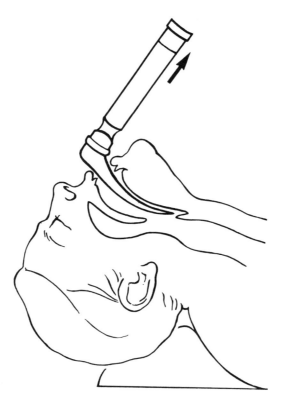

Fig. 6.5 Direct laryngoscopy

It is important to note that the laryngoscope should be lifted in the direction that the handle is pointing and not levered by movement of the wrist, as this might damage the teeth and will not provide as good a view.

The tracheal tube should be introduced from the right-hand side of the mouth and inserted between the vocal cords into the larynx under direct vision. Once the tube is in place, the cuff should be inflated just sufficiently to provide an air-tight seal between the tube and the trachea. A catheter mount is then attached to the tube and ventilation commenced. Checks should then be made to ensure correct positioning of the tube and confirm ventilation of both lungs, by looking for bilateral chest movement with ventilation, listening for breath sounds bilaterally in the mid-axillary line and finally listening for gurgling sounds over the epigastrium, which may indicate inadvertent oesophageal intubation. The ultimate check for correct placement of the tube is measurement of carbon dioxide in the expired gas, which will be <0.1% in any gas coming back out of the stomach, indicating oesophageal placement of the tube.

Tracheal intubation is not without risks. All the structures encountered from the lips to the trachea may be traumatized and when the degree of unconsciousness has been misjudged, vomiting may be stimulated. The use of a tube that is too long may result in it passing into a main bronchus (usually the right), causing the opposite lung to collapse, thereby severely impairing the efficiency of ventilation. As the average distance between the incisors and carina is 27 cm in the adult male and 23 cm in the female, oral tubes need to be 23 cm long for males and 21 cm long for females (add 4 cm for nasal intubation). The most dangerous problem associated with tracheal intubation is unrecognized oesophageal intubation. The patient may appear to be ventilating adequately, but in fact is receiving no oxygen at all and rapidly becoming hypoxic. **If in doubt, take it out!** and ventilate the patient using a bag–valve–mask.

Tracheal intubation is frequently more difficult to perform during resuscitation. The patient may be awkwardly positioned on the floor, equipment may be unfamiliar, assistance limited, CPR obstructive and vomit copious. In these circumstances, it is all too easy to persist with the 'almost there' attitude. This must be strongly resisted and if intubation is not successfully accomplished in approximately 30–40 s (about the time one can breath-hold during the attempt), it should be abandoned and ventilation with 100% oxygen using a bag–valve–mask should recommence before and in-between any further attempts at intubation.

Occasionally, direct pressure from an assistant on the thyroid cartilage may aid visualization of the cords (not to be confused with cricoid pressure), particularly when the larynx is very anterior. In a small percentage of patients, only the very posterior part of the cords (or none) can be seen and passage of the tracheal tube becomes difficult. In these cases, a gum-elastic introducer can initially be inserted into the larynx and then the tube slid over the introducer into the larynx. However, it must be remembered that the patient must be oxygenated in-between attempts at intubation.

6.2.2 Cricoid pressure (Figure 6.6)

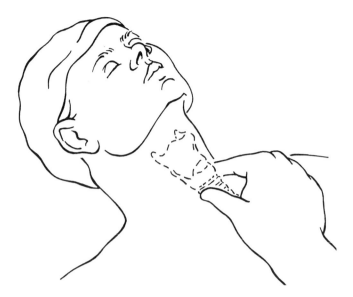

Fig. 6.6 Technique for cricoid pressure

This is a manoeuvre used by anaesthetists who employ it to prevent regurgitation of gastric contents into the lungs during the induction of anaesthesia in patients with a full stomach. Pressure is applied on the **cricoid cartilage** by an assistant, thereby compressing the oesophagus against the body of the sixth cervical vertebra. This prevents passive regurgitation, but should not be used during active vomiting. If incorrectly applied, it may make intubation more difficult.

6.2.3 Ventilation

Whichever technique is used to ventilate the patient, the ultimate aim is to increase the inspired oxygen concentration to 100%. The most common device used to ventilate patients who are apnoeic or breathing inadequately is the self-inflating bag (Ambu or Laerdal type). This can be connected via a non-rebreathing valve to either a face-mask or a tracheal tube. Used alone, this will allow ventilation of the patient with 21% oxygen as it refills with ambient air. However this concentration can (and should) be increased during resuscitation, firstly to 50% by connecting an oxygen supply at 6 l/min directly to the bag adjacent to the air intake, and then to 95% by supplying oxygen to a reservoir bag from which the bag refills (Figure 6.7).

Although the self-inflating bag and valve are widely used they are associated with several problems. When attached to a face-mask it requires considerable skill to apply the mask, maintain a gas-tight seal with the face and lift the jaw with one hand while squeezing the bag with the other hand. In addition, gas may pass into the stomach, resulting in hypoventilation and gastric dilatation. The valve mechanism may become blocked with

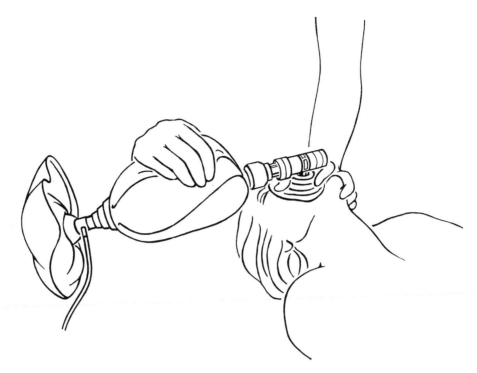

Fig. 6.7 Self-inflating bag and mask with reservoir

secretions and is susceptible to heavy moisture contamination, causing it to stick. If the bag is used without a reservoir, oxygen delivery is not optimal for resuscitation. The latter two problems apply equally when this system is being used to ventilate a patient via a tracheal tube. They can be overcome to some extent by using a catheter mount between the tube and valve and a reservoir bag to ensure delivery of the highest concentration of oxygen.

Another method used to ventilate patients, either via a face-mask or tube, is the Waters Circuit (Mapleson C, Westminster Face-piece or rebreathing bag). In this system, the bag fills by a combination of the oxygen flowing into it and the expired air from the patient. An adjustable expiratory valve is also provided. By almost completely closing the expiratory valve, it appears possible to ventilate patients adequately with a low flow of oxygen (4 l/min), as judged by breath sounds and chest movement. However, unless a high flow of oxygen (12–15 l/min) is used to flush the system, expired air (containing 5% carbon dioxide) accumulates within the bag and the patient rebreaths (or is ventilated) with expired gas and rapidly becomes hypercarbic. This situation is particularly dangerous to any patient who has raised intracranial pressure from whatever cause. Because of this potential danger and the inefficiency of this system, it should not be used during resuscitation.

The ultimate method of ventilating patients during resuscitation is with a mechanical ventilator. The most important feature of these devices is that they are good servants, but poor masters – they will only do what they are set to do. Therefore it is imperative that they are set correctly when used. Portable ventilators are generally gas powered. The relevance of this is that, when using an oxygen cylinder as both the power supply and the source of respiratory gas for the patient, the cylinder will be used up more rapidly. Care must be taken to ensure adequate oxygen supplies during the transport of ventilated patients over long distances.

Pneumatic portable ventilators are classified as time cycled, with a fixed inspiratory:expiratory ratio. They provide a constant flow of gas during inspiration and therefore deliver a preset tidal volume. As a safety feature, they can be pressure limited. This limits the tidal volume if a predetermined pressure is reached during inspiration, thereby protecting the lungs against baro-trauma. Expiration occurs passively to the atmosphere. When using a ventilator, it should be set to deliver a tidal volume of 10–15 ml/kg at a rate of 12 breaths per minute. Many ventilators have co-ordinated markings around the controls to facilitate rapid easy setting, for different sized patients. The correct setting of ventilatory parameters ultimately depends upon the result of analysis of arterial blood gases.

6.2.4 The surgical airway

Occasionally, ventilation of a patient will not be possible using any of the techniques described so far. This is usually due to obstruction of the airway either above the vocal cords or within the larynx, most commonly caused by the presence of a foreign body. Other causes are trauma, local inflammation or tumour. Under these circumstances, when all other means have failed, it will be necessary to create a surgical airway below the level of the obstruction.

Needle cricothyroidotomy and cricothyroidotomy are covered in Annex B.

Annex A
Equipment and technique for tracheal intubation

EQUIPMENT

1. Laryngoscope: most commonly with a curved (Macintosh) blade
2. Tracheal tubes: females 7.5–8.0 mm internal diameter, 21 cm long; males 8.0–9.0 mm internal diameter, 23 cm long
3. Syringe, to inflate the cuff
4. Catheter mount, to attach to ventilating device
5. Lubricant, for tube, water-soluble, preferably sterile
6. Magills forceps
7. Introducers, malleable and gum elastic, for difficult cases
8. Adhesive tapes or bandages for securing tube
9. Ventilator
10. Suction

TECHNIQUE

1. Check equipment function, particularly: laryngoscope, suction, ventilation device
2. Choose correct size tracheal tube: length, diameter, cuff integrity
3. Preoxygenate the patient
4. Correct positioning of head
5. Laryngoscopy: holding laryngoscope correctly
6. Intubation: accomplished in <35 s for adults and <30 s in children from 'mask off'. In the event of failure, re-establish ventilation with bag–valve–mask
7. Correct attachment of ventilating device
8. Ability to check correct positioning of tracheal tube and sequence of events if negative

Annex B
Needle cricothyroidotomy and cricothyroidotomy

It is important to realize that these techniques are temporizing measures, while preparations are made to provide a definitive airway.

NEEDLE CRICOTHYROIDOTOMY (FIGURE 6.8)

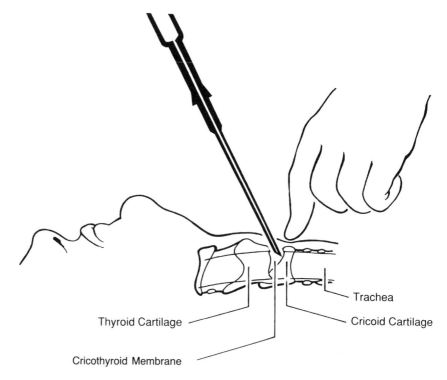

Fig. 6.8 Needle cricothyroid-otomy

Thyroid Cartilage

Cricothyroid Membrane

Trachea

Cricoid Cartilage

The cricothyroid membrane is identified as the recessed area between the thyroid cartilage (Adam's apple), and the next lower solid bar of cartilage, the cricoid cartilage. It is approximately 2 cm below the 'V' shaped notch of the thyroid cartilage. This membrane (or the trachea below the cricoid cartilage) is punctured vertically with a large bore (12 g or 14 g) cannula. Aspiration of air usually indicates correct placement. The cannula is then angulated to 45°, advanced down the trachea and connected to an oxygen source at 15 l/min via a 'Y' connector (or a side hole should be cut in the delivery tubing). Oxygen is then delivered to the patient by intermittently covering the hole for 1 s followed by 4 s off. An alternative method is to use jet ventilation. This involves connecting the cannula to a high-pressure oxygen supply (4 bar, 60 psi), using a Sanders injector. The same ventilatory cycle is used. Once ventilation commences, the chest should be observed for movement, and auscultated for breath sounds. The cannula should then be secured to prevent it being dislodged.

Although needle cricothyroidotomy allows oxygenation of the patient, carbon dioxide is not eliminated efficiently and therefore the usefulness of this technique is limited to about 45 min. As the larynx may be partially occluded, it is essential to allow sufficient time for expiration to occur. Failure to do so can lead to progressively higher intrathoracic pressures which will embarrass venous return and cardiac output and cause pulmonary damage and pneumothoraces. Other complications of this technique include bleeding, oesophageal perforation and kinking of the cannula. If the cannula is inadvertently positioned in the soft tissues anteriorly to the trachea, ventilation can result in the rapid development of subcutaneous and mediastinal emphysema. In some instances, this method of ventilation may disimpact a foreign body from the larynx, allowing resumption of more acceptable methods.

CRICOTHYROIDOTOMY (FIGURE 6.9)

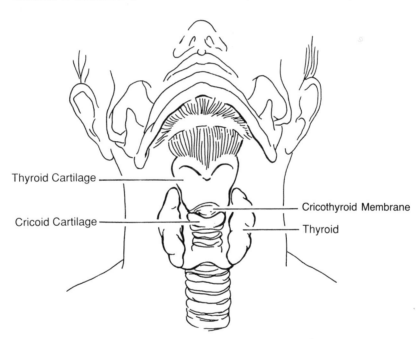

Fig. 6.9 Cricothyroid-otomy, relevant anatomy

Thyroid Cartilage

Cricoid Cartilage

Cricothyroid Membrane

Thyroid

Again, this is an emergency measure, not a definitive airway. The technique consists of identifying the cricothyroid membrane as above. The thyroid cartilage is then stabilized using the thumb, index and middle fingers of the left hand while making an incision through the cricothyroid membrane. The opening is then dilated to accept either a small (4–7 mm) tracheal or tracheostomy tube. Ideally a purpose-designed kit should be used (in an emergency, any strong, sharp instrument, e.g. scissors can suffice). When a cuffed tube has been inserted, the cuff should be inflated and ventilation commenced. Once again, adequacy of ventilation should be confirmed by observation and auscultation of the chest and the tube should be secured. Because a large-diameter airway is created, effective artificial ventilation can be performed, allowing both oxygenation and elimination of carbon dioxide. In addition a fine suction catheter (no longer than half the diameter of the tube) can be passed into the airway to remove any debris, blood or secretions.

A recent development which has proved useful in these circumstances is the 'Mini-Trach' (Portex). Although originally designed to facilitate removal of secretions from the chest, the kit contains all the bits and pieces needed to create an emergency surgical airway. A guarded scalpel is used to puncture the cricothyroid membrane percutaneously. A rigid, curved introducer is then passed through the puncture site into the trachea. A 4 mm PVC tracheal cannula is then passed over the introducer into the trachea. The introducer is removed and the cannula secured. A 4 mm Portex connector can be used to permit ventilation using standard equipment.

Complications are similar to needle cricothyroidotomy, except that bleeding can be more severe due to the larger incision. In the long term hoarseness can result from damage to the vocal cords and laryngeal stenosis can result from damage to the cricoid cartilage.

Practical skill station
Adult and paediatric airway

AIMS

To reinforce practically the knowledge of airway control and ventilation gained during theoretical sessions.

To allow candidates to demonstrate proficiency in airway control and ventilation using both an adult and paediatric airway management manikin.

TEACHING TECHNIQUE

Candidates are given a practical demonstration by instructors and are then given the opportunity to practice the procedures using the airway management manikins.

TESTING

Candidates are assessed informally on their performance during this skill station. On testing day, candidates are expected to demonstrate their ability to manage the airway and ventilate both the adult and paediatric manikins successfully.

Practical skill station
Adult and paediatric intubation

AIMS

To apply practically the knowledge of intubation gained in theoretical sessions.

To allow candidates to demonstrate their ability to intubate both the adult and paediatric manikins.

TEACHING TECHNIQUE

Candidates are given a practical demonstration by instructors and are then given the opportunity to practice the procedures using the airway management manikins.

TESTING

Candidates are assessed informally on their performance during this skill station. On testing day, candidates are expected to demonstrate their ability to intubate both the adult and paediatric manikins successfully.

7

Monitoring and dysrhythmia recognition

Objectives

After studying this chapter you should be able to:

- Understand the components of an ECG rhythm strip

- Understand how the cardiac rhythm can be monitored

- Understand a system of rhythm strip analysis

- Recognize the immediately and potentially life-threatening dysrhythmias

- Demonstrate proficiency at dysrhythmia recognition using rhythm strips and 12-lead ECGs

- Given a simulated patient model, demonstrate proficiency at dysrhythmia recognition during resuscitation

This chapter is designed to enable the reader to understand and recognize the dysrhythmias presented. It is not aimed at replacing the many excellent ECG books currently on the market.

7.1 ANATOMY OF THE NORMAL CONDUCTION SYSTEM

In the normal state, the stimulation for cardiac contraction originates in a specialized area of cardiac muscle called the sino-atrial (S-A) node. The electrical impulse then radiates through the right and left atrial muscles inducing contraction. This electrical wave gives rise to the 'P' wave on the ECG, with both atria acting together to produce a single P wave (Figure 7.1).

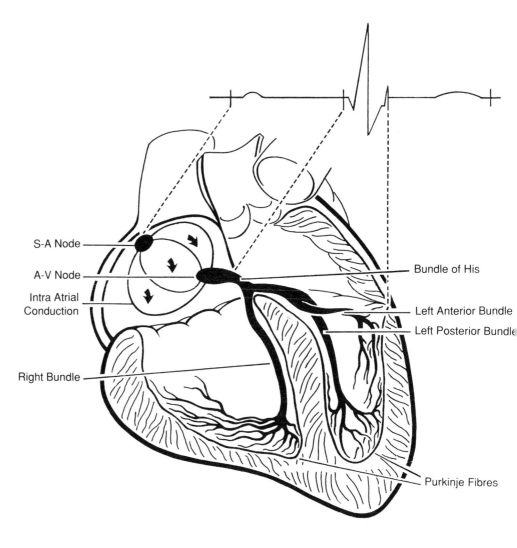

Fig. 7.1 The conduction system of the heart and its relationship to the ECG

S-A Node

A-V Node

Intra Atrial Conduction

Right Bundle

Bundle of His

Left Anterior Bundle

Left Posterior Bundle

Purkinje Fibres

The atria and ventricles are separated by a fibrous barrier which blocks the transmission of the electrical impulse. Normally, the only breach in this barrier is at the atrio-ventricular (A-V) node which is located in the base of the right atria. Conduction of the impulse to the ventricles therefore occurs via the A-V node once it has been stimulated by the electrical impulse spreading through the atria. The higher resistance to conduction in the A-V node results in a delay in this transmission and is the main cause, on the ECG, for the PR interval. This time period is measured from the start of the P wave to the first deflection of the QRS complex.

Electrical conduction in the ventricles is initially by specialized muscle bundles. The Bundle of His is located in the proximal part of the septum. Distally, it splits into the right and left bundle, the latter subsequently separating into the anterior and posterior divisions (fascicles). These specialized bundles terminate in small (Purkinje) fibres which transmit the electrical impulse to the non-specialized ventricular myocardium. The passage of the impulse through the ventricle is demonstrated by the QRS wave on the ECG.

Following stimulation, the myocardial cells recover their normal resting electrical potential in an active biochemical process called repolarization. The atrial repolarization wave is usually obscured by the QRS, but the ventricular repolarization gives rise to the ST segment and the T wave. This is sometimes followed by a U wave, which is a rounded deflection in the same direction as the T wave. Its origin is unclear but it becomes more prominent in hypokalaemia and inverted in ischaemic heart disease.

The QT interval is measured from the beginning of the QRS complex to the end of the T wave. Normally it is 0.35–0.42 s, but its duration is inversely dependent on the heart rate, and directly dependent on age and sex.

A summation of all the electrical impulses in the heart produces the cardiac axis. As seen from the front, this runs from 11 o'clock to 5 o'clock. This direction results from the large left ventricular muscle mass. For further details on how to determine the cardiac axis, the interested reader should consult Annex A at the end of this chapter.

7.2 GENERAL RULES IN MONITORING THE CARDIAC RHYTHM

7.2.1 Theory

The ECG monitor should be used in all cases presenting with chest pain, syncope, dizziness, collapse, palpitations and cardiac arrest.

ECG machines run at a standard speed of 25 mm/s. Calibrated recording paper is used so that each large square is equivalent to 0.2 s and each small square to 0.04 s. The amplitude of the trace is standardized at 1 mV per cm. Most machines have the capability of testing this (Figure 7.2).

Fig. 7.2
Voltage
calibration

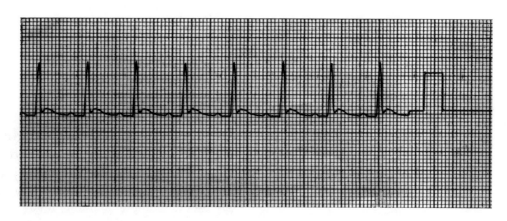

The electrodes monitor the electrical conduction through the heart. For each lead, the electrical activity is measured between two 'active' electrodes with a third acting as a 'ground' or reference electrode. If the impulse is moving towards the electrode then an upward or positive deflection is seen on the monitor. Conversely, if the impulse moves away from the electrode then a downward or 'negative' deflection is seen on the monitor.

The electrodes view the electrical activity of the heart either in the vertical or horizontal plane. Leads I, II, III, and AVR, AVL, AVF look at the heart in the vertical plane. Leads V1–6, also known as the 'chest leads', view the heart in the horizontal plane. Dysrhythmia analysis concentrates mainly on those leads viewing the electrical activity in the vertical plane.

Lead I measures the voltage between the right and left shoulder with the left lower chest electrode being the ground electrode. It gives a good view of the left lateral aspect of the heart and the QRS complex (Figure 7.3). It does not necessarily give a good picture of the P wave.

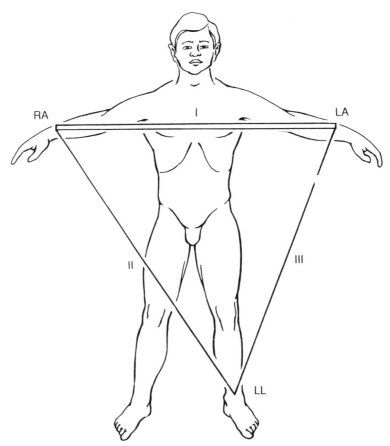

Fig. 7.3 The bipolar limb leads

Lead II measures the voltage between the right shoulder and left lower chest. It is in line with the cardiac axis (running approximately from 11 o'clock to 5 o'clock) and consequently gives a good view of both the QRS and P wave (Figure 7.3). It will also show shifts in the direction of the cardiac axis in left axis deviation (see Annex A). It is the lead most commonly used for monitoring the cardiac rhythm.

Lead III measures the voltage between the left shoulder and left lower chest. It is rarely an advantage in dysrhythmia recognition but it does give a good view of the inferior aspect of the heart (Figure 7.3).

The remaining leads are not used during a cardiac arrest. They are, however, required for definitive dysrhythmia analysis as they give views of particular parts of the heart. They are also needed to determine the position of the cardiac axis (see Annex A for details).

The standard leads view the heart vertically from either the left, right or anterior aspects (Figure 7.4).

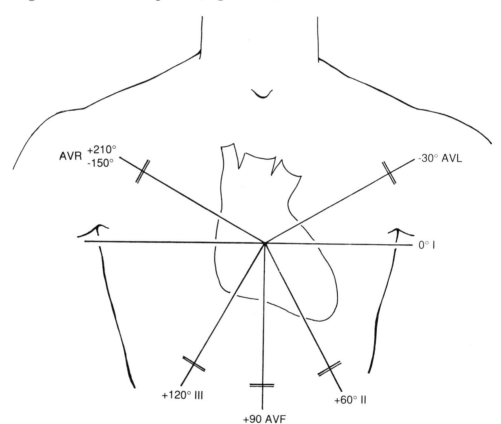

Fig. 7.4 The standard lead view of the heart

V1 and V2 view the right side of the heart, V3 and V4 the septum and V5 and V6, mainly the left ventricle (Figure 7.5).

If the QRS complexes from the chest leads are grouped together, the R wave can be seen to get gradually bigger as one reads from 1 to 6, and the P and S waves gradually smaller. The T wave is usually upright in all the chest leads (Figure 7.6).

73

Fig. 7.5   The chest leads

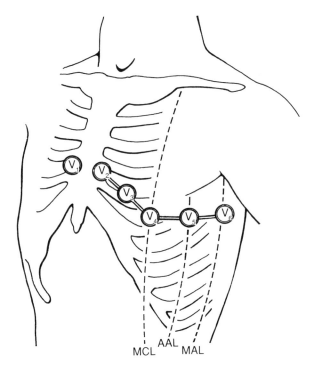

**Fig. 7.6
Normal R wave progression**

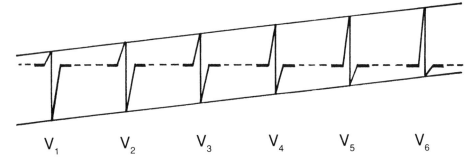

In V1 and V2 the P wave can be inverted or biphasic, the T waves inverted and the Q wave larger than two small squares in depth and 0.04 s in duration.

The MCL1 lead measures the voltage between the left shoulder and the right pectoral area. This gives a good view of the QRS and P wave, but it is not commonly used outside coronary care units.

The leads used to monitor dysrhythmias are not the optimum ones for recording changes in the ST segment and T wave. A 'diagnostic' setting may be required to reproduce ST displacement accurately, but this produces more baseline wandering.

7.2.2 Practical points

To minimize interference, the electrodes should be all of the same type, applied over bone rather than muscle and positioned such that the ground electrode is equidistant between the two active electrodes.

The electrodes should be attached to the patient's chest so that they will not interfere with any other activities, such as external cardiac massage.

Adhesive silver/silver chloride electrodes give the best signal and, if readily available, are preferable to defibrillation paddles even for the first 'quick look' in cardiac arrest. In addition, paddles will only give a reading when they are in position, and so they are not practical for assessing the rhythm continuously. If paddles are used, it is essential that gel pads are used to facilitate electrical contact.

Ensure that the QRS height is sufficient to stimulate the rate metre, by adjusting the gain control, but not so excessive as to cause artefacts on the monitor.

Any activity, such as drug administration or carotid sinus massage, should be recorded on the rhythm strip as it happens. This helps greatly in the later analysis of the dysrhythmia.

If time permits, a full 12 lead ECG should be carried out as this facilitates dysrhythmia analysis. However, during a cardiac arrest, the use of lead II is usually sufficient.

7.3 PATHOLOGY OF THE CONDUCTING SYSTEM

The electrical conduction through the heart can be blocked at various places, from ischaemic disease, drugs, trauma and abnormal metabolic conditions.

Sino-atrial block prevents the sinus impulse depolarizing the atria but does not reset the S-A node timer. As a consequence, no P waves are produced while the block is present but, when it stops, P waves return at a multiple of the normal PP interval (Figure 7.7).

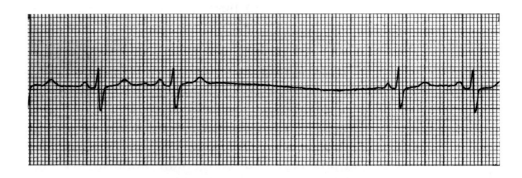

Fig. 7.7 Sino-atrial block

Sinus arrest is when the S-A node is no longer functioning. If this, or sinus block, does not spontaneously rectify, another part of the heart will have to take over as the pacemaker. All parts of the special conducting system have the ability to initiate an electrical impulse but do so at varying frequencies. The eventual heart rate is determined by that part of the conducting system which has the fastest intrinsic rate of impulse production. Normally this is the S-A node, but following damage the next fastest part of the system takes over as the cardiac pacemaker. This is usually the atrial muscles, followed by the A-V node, Bundle of His and eventually the ventricular myocardium.

Blockage and conduction delays can also occur in the A-V node, Bundle of His, right and left bundle and the anterior and posterior fascicle, either separately or in combination. Though their causes are similar, their treatment and prognosis can be quite different. The ECG can be used to distinguish between them.

Occasionally a pathological focus develops, in the atria or ventricles, which has a faster rate of impulse production than the S-A node. This will then replace the S-A node as the cardiac pacemaker.

7.4 CAUSES OF DYSRHYTHMIA

7.4.1 Slowing of the heart rate

A slow heart rate is a normal physiological response during sleep and at rest in the athletic individual. In the pathological situation a slow heart rate can also be produced, but this results from damage to the conducting system. Ischaemic heart disease is the most common cause but drugs, trauma and other disease can also be responsible.

7.4.2 Increasing of the heart rate

An increase in heart rate occurs normally as a result of emotion, exercise and fear. It can also occur for the following pathological reasons:

1. **Automaticity**: This is when a specific area of the conducting system, or myocardium, increases its rate of spontaneous discharge or depolarization. If this is faster than the S-A node rate then it becomes the new cardiac pacemaker.
2. **Re-entry**: This occurs when there is a dual conducting system from either a congenital abnormality (e.g. Wolfe–Parkinson–White, see Annex B) or ischaemic heart disease. One pathway (A) has a unidirectional block (or a longer refractory period) and the other (B) has a slow conduction rate (Figure 7.8).

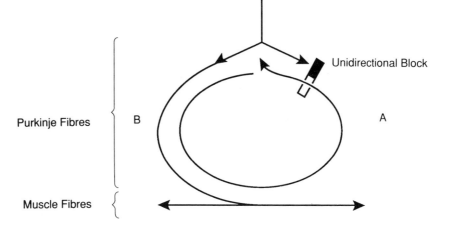

Fig. 7.8 The origin of a circus movement

Purkinje Fibres

Muscle Fibres

B

A

Unidirectional Block

In response to a premature beat, the impulse has to go down the slow pathway (B) because the fast pathway (A) is still refractory from the previous beat. This increase in transit time allows A to recover so that the impulse can be conducted in a retrograde fashion, back into the atria. By this time, B has recovered and so can be stimulated by this re-entry impulse.

3. **Both**: Automaticity and re-entry can act together.

Unless there is an extra systole before the tachycardia commences, it is not possible on the surface ECG to distinguish between enhanced automaticity and re-entry.

7.5 DYSRHYTHMIA RECOGNITION

Always remember: treat the patient not the rhythm

Avoid the temptation to simply 'eye ball' the strip. Instead go through the whole rhythm strip in a methodical manner so that clues and multiple problems are not missed.

Listed below are a series of questions which need to be answered before a dysrhythmia diagnosis can be made.

1. Is there any electrical activity at all?

If not, check:

Connections
QRS gain
Leads I and III

If there is still no electrical activity, diagnose asystole (see Figure 7.9).

Fig. 7.9
Asystole

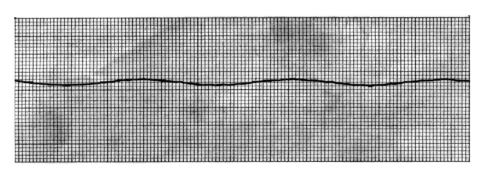

There are two types – those with P waves and those without. The former has the better prognosis.

Beware that a completely flat trace, without any baseline wandering, is usually caused by the patient's leads not being connected to the monitor.

2. Are there any recognizable complexes?

If there are no recognizable complexes, diagnose ventricular fibrillation (VF) (Figure 7.10).

Fig. 7.10 Ventricular fibrillation

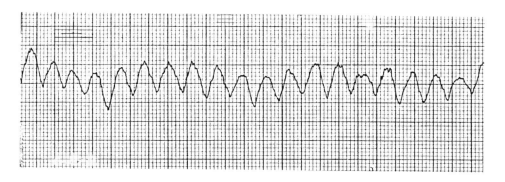

This gives rise to a totally chaotic rhythm because individual muscle fibres are contracting independently. Initially, the complexes are large and the dysrhythmia is known as coarse VF. Over time, these diminish and the tracing becomes flatter. This is called fine VF.

VF is the commonest cause of cardiac arrest in ischaemic heart disease.

If there are recognizable complexes:

3. What is the ventricular rate?

$$\text{Rate} = \frac{300}{\text{No. of large squares between consecutive R waves}} \quad (7.1)$$

Figure 7.11 shows a ventricular rate of 75 beats/min.

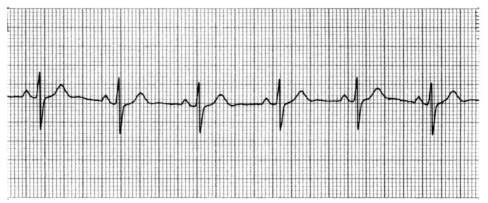

Fig. 7.11 Sinus rhythm: rate 75 beats/min

A ventricular rate greater than 100 beats/min is called a tachycardia.

Sinus tachycardia has a P wave before each QRS and usually has a rate of 100–130 beats/min (Figure 7.12).

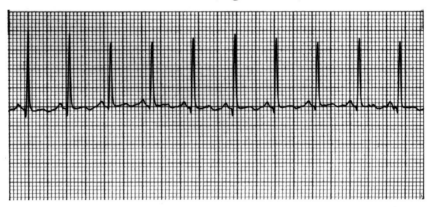

Fig. 7.12 Sinus tachycardia: rate 136 beats/min

Supraventricular tachycardia (SVT) can be divided into two types:

(i) Paroxysmal SVT. 'Paroxysmal' indicates that the dysrhythmia is self-terminating. This type of SVT produces a regular ventricular rhythm of 150 beats/min or higher and it is usually due to the re-entry phenomenon mentioned in Section 7.4.2 (Figure 7.13).

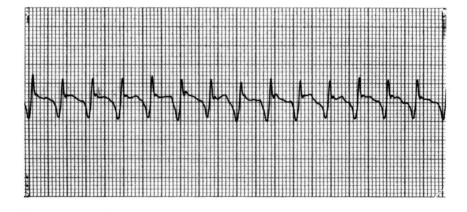

Fig. 7.13 Paroxysmal SVT

The QRS complexes are narrow unless there is an aberrant conduction through the Bundle of His producing widening of the QRS complex. Commonly, this type of dysrhythmia has a sudden onset.

(ii) Non-paroxysmal SVT. This produces an irregular ventricular rhythm of between 60 and 150 beats/min, usually as a result of altered automaticity.

A ventricular rate of less than 60 beats/min is called a bradycardia.

Sinus bradycardia also has a P wave before each QRS. It is common after inferior infarction.

4. What is the rhythm?

P waves have a duration of 0.08–0.12 s (2–3 small squares) and a deflection less than 2.5 mm in height. They can be distinguished from the larger T wave which has a duration of 0.28 s.

It is important to check the whole strip for P waves because they may be hidden in the QRS complex or T wave, producing abnormal 'lumps and bumps' (Figure 7.14).

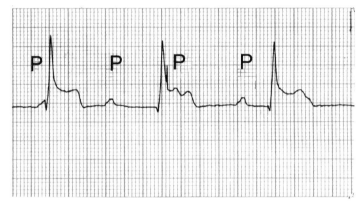

Fig. 7.14 P waves hidden in the QRS complex

Occasionally, hidden P waves can be revealed by slowing the ventricular rate by either carotid sinus massage or drugs.

If P waves are present and precede each QRS complex, and successive RR intervals are regular, then this is known as a sinus rhythm. Occasionally in healthy young individuals, the RR interval varies with respiration but the P wave shape and PR interval remain constant. During inspiration the heart rate increases as a result of vagal impulses inhibiting the cardioinhibitory centre. The opposite occurs during expiration. This variation in rate is called sinus arrhythmia.

If there are no P waves then an assessment of the regularity of the rhythm of the R waves must be made. An accurate way of doing this is to mark the peaks of four R waves on a piece of paper. This must be done precisely because rhythm irregularity becomes less marked as the heart rate speeds up. The paper is then moved along the strip to see if the RR gaps correspond. The absence of any pattern is known as an 'irregular irregularity'.

When this rhythm is associated with a narrow QRS complex (i.e. less than or equal to 0.12 s), a diagnosis of atrial fibrillation (AF) can be made (Figure 7.15).

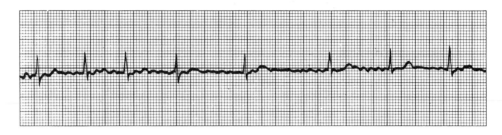

Fig. 7.15 Atrial fibrillation

There are no P waves with AF, but the baseline may vary between fine and course fluctuations in different parts of the strip.

AF is due to atrial depolarization in a disorganized fashion at a rate of 300–500/min with conduction through the A-V node occurring at an irregular rate.

5. Are the P waves of uniform shape?

Abnormally shaped P waves do not originate from the S-A node. They have two possible sources:

(i) Ectopic focus. This usually originates in the atria, rarely from the A-V node. These are known as atrial and junctional extra systoles, respectively. If the source is from the atria then the P wave is upright in lead II, i.e. the impulse is still moving towards that electrode. If the source is the A-V node, then the P wave may be buried in the QRS or T wave. The other distinguishing feature of ectopic foci is the PPi interval, i.e the time period between the normal P wave and the ectopic. This is **shorter** than that between two normal P waves (PP) because the ectopic focus is sending out its electrical impulses at a faster rate than the S-A node (Figure 7.16).

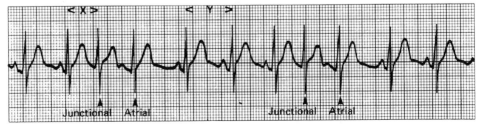

Fig. 7.16 Ectopic P waves. Note PP (Y) and PPi (X) intervals

The ectopic P wave (shown in Figure 7.12) blocks the S-A node from discharging and so disturbs the rhythm of P wave production. This can be demonstrated on the rhythm strip by noting the interval between the normal P waves on either side of the ectopic beat. This distance is not equal to twice the normal PP interval.

The focus may only produce one abnormal P wave. Alternatively it may take over completely and so not allow any normal (S-A node-generated) P waves to occur for a prolonged period of time. The whole rhythm strip will need to be studied to determine if a normal PP interval can be found.

The coupling interval is a term used to describe the distance between a normal P wave and P'. This is constant if the ectopic is always produced from the same focus.

(ii) Escape beat (see Figure 7.17). If the S-A node fails to send out its electrical impulse then another part of the conduction system will fire off instead. This is known as an escape beat. As described above, it is the atrial muscles followed by the A-V node which take over as the cardiac pacemaker in this situation. The escape beat can be distinguished by two features:

1. The PP interval between normal and escape P wave is **longer** than the normal (S-A node-generated) PP interval.
2. The escape P wave is either inverted because the impulse is moving away from lead II (shown in Figure 7.17) or is hidden in the QRS/T wave.

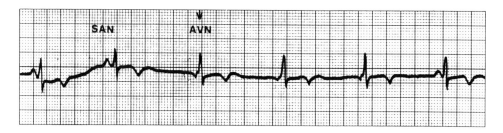

Fig. 7.17 Escape P waves

Atrial escape beats may be sustained with each impulse coming from a different part of the atria, and a constantly changing P wave morphology and PR interval results. This condition is known as a wandering atrial pacemaker.

6. Is there atrial flutter?

In atrial flutter (Figure 7.18), the atrial muscles are depolarizing at 300 beats/min. This characteristically produces a 'saw-tooth' appearance in leads II, III and AVF.

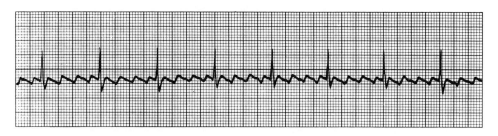

Fig. 7.18 Atrial flutter

As the A-V node has a longer refractory period than the atria, there is a block to the atrial impulses. Consequently, only one in two or one in four get through to the ventricles. However the QRS complexes which result will have a normal shape because this part of the conduction system has not been altered.

7. Are the number of P and QRS waves the same?

Again, study the whole rhythm strip to make sure P waves are not hidden in the QRS or T waves. If the number of P and QRS waves are the same, look then at the PR interval (1 small square is 0.04 s):

Less than 0.12 s: nodal rhythm, Wolfe–Parkinson–White, Lown–Ganong–Levine (see Annex B)
0.12–0.2 s: sinus rhythm
Over 0.2 s: first degree heart block

The latter is shown in Figure 7.19. It is an ECG diagnosis and generally does not progress to more serious forms of heart block. It is asymptomatic.

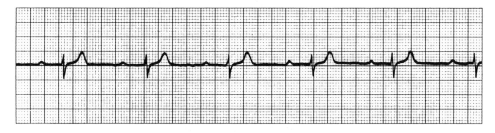

Fig. 7.19 First degree block

If the number of P waves is greater than the number of QRS waves then the patient has either second or third degree heart block. To distinguish between them the PR interval must be examined.

There are two varieties of second degree heart block.

(i) Mobitz Type I (Wenkebach) (Figure 7.20).

Fig. 7.20
Second degree
block – Mobitz
type I

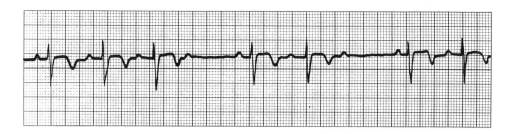

In this condition the PR interval progressively lengthens, until a P wave does not propagate a QRS complex. The AVN then recovers and the next PR interval reverts to the previous shortest conduction time. This rhythm is therefore distinguished by having **both varying PR and RR intervals**. This is a transient phenomenon and is commonly found following inferior myocardial infarction.

(ii) Mobitz Type II (Figure 7.21).

Fig. 7.21
Second degree
block – Mobitz
type II

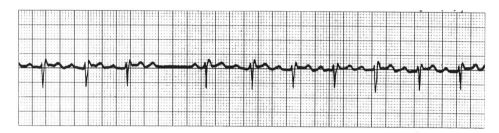

In this condition there is an intermittent non-conduction of some P waves but **the PR interval remains constant**. This dysrhythmia is much more likely to progress to third degree heart block than Type I and there is a higher chance of developing asystole or ventricular dysrhythmias. This condition is associated with anterior myocardial infarction. The QRS complexes are usually broad due to abnormal ventricular conduction.

In third degree or complete heart block there is total dissociation between the depolarization of atria and ventricles with each beating independently (Figure 7.22). As a consequence, there is no relationship between P waves and the QRS complexes on the ECG trace. The PR interval is therefore completely erratic **but the PP and RR intervals are constant**.

Fig. 7.22   Third
degree (complete)
block

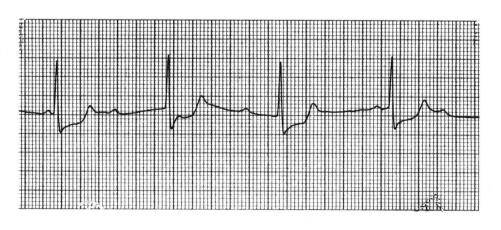

The QRS complex can be narrow or wide depending on where the source of the ventricular pacemaker is located. A focus near the A-V node will result in a rate of around 50 beats/min with narrow complexes as they are conducted via the Bundle of His. This is associated with an inferior myocardial infarction.

A ventricular focus, which is more distal, will produce a rate of around 30 beats/min with wide QRS complexes because conduction through the ventricles is not by the normal pathway. This is associated with an anterior myocardial infarction or marked ischaemic heart disease. These patients have a worse prognosis than those with a narrow QRS.

8. Is the QRS duration normal?

The normal duration for the QRS is 0.12 s (3 small squares) or less. Broader complexes occur as a result of:

(i) Ventricular ectopic beats. These beats originate from an unstable area of the ventricular myocardium. They are not usually conducted through the Bundle of His, therefore a widened, slow complex is produced (see Figure 7.23). Depolarization is premature, thereby reducing the interval between the normal and abnormal beats (RR'). There is also no proceeding P wave because it is buried in the abnormal QRS complex.

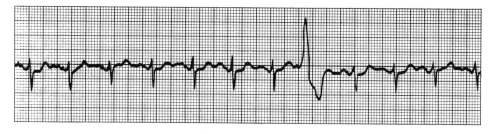

Fig. 7.23
Ventricular ectopic

These ectopic impulses do not alter, or reset, the S-A node. Therefore the frequency of P waves will continue undisturbed by the abnormal ventricular activity with the next P wave occurring at the normal time. Compare this with the atrial ectopic beat described previously.

Particular emphasis is placed on the ventricular ectopic which occurs close to the T wave. It is stated that there is a higher chance of precipitating ventricular fibrillation if the ectopic fires during the repolarization phase of the ventricle. This is known as the R-on-T phenomenon (Figure 7.24).

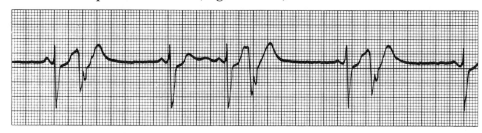

Fig. 7.24   R-on-T ectopic

When there is more than one ventricular ectopic, specific terms are used:

(ii) Multifocal ventricular ectopics. The ectopic varies in shape from beat to beat when there is more than one source (see Figure 7.25).

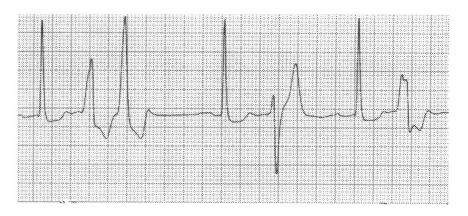

Fig. 7.25 Multifocal ventricular ectopics

(iii) Bigemini. The ventricular ectopic is followed by a normal QRS (Figure 7.26).

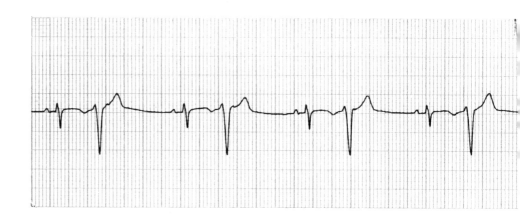

Fig. 7.26 Bigemini

(iv) Trigemini. When the ventricular ectopic is followed by two normal QRS complexes (Figure 7.27).

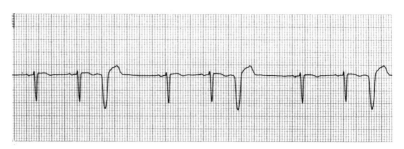

Fig. 7.27 Trigemini

(v) Couplet. There are two ventricular ectopic beats in a row (Figure 7.28).

(vi) Ventricular tachycardia: There are three or more ectopic beats in a row (see later).

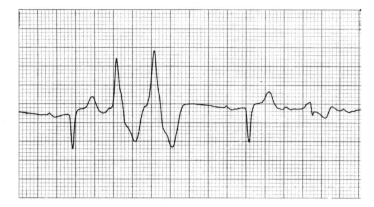

Fig. 7.28 Couplets

(vii) Ventricular escape beats. These occur when the S-A and A-V nodes can no longer generate an electrical impulse or stimulate the ventricles. The heart rate is slow and the RR interval is longer than normal. If P waves exist they do not have any connection to the QRS.

(viii) Aberrant conduction with supraventricular ectopic stimulation. The QRS is abnormal because the ectopic impulse gets to either the ventricles or A-V node before they have had a chance to repolarize fully from the preceding stimulation. This results in a right bundle branch block pattern or a complete block at the A-V node. Occasionally the shape of the QRS varies from beat to beat because the conduction pathway through the ventricles is not consistent. The PR interval is normal or slightly prolonged.

(ix) Intraventricular bundle branch block. This occurs when either the right or left bundle cannot conduct the electrical impulse. A 12-lead ECG is required to make the diagnosis.

In left bundle branch block, most of the tracing looks abnormal. The QRS complexes are wider than 0.12 s, there is a small R in V1 (QrS) and a characteristic 'M' shaped QRS complex in V6 (rsR'). In the lateral leads (1, AVL, V5, V6) the Q and S waves are absent, and there may be associated ST depression and T wave inversion (Figure 7.29).

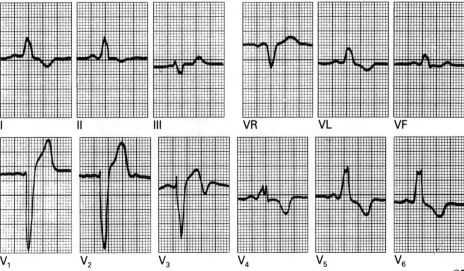

Fig. 7.29 Left bundle branch block

Right bundle branch block gives rise to a wide (>0.12 s) QRS with a tall, secondary R in lead V1. This is known as an rsR′ pattern (Figure 7.30).

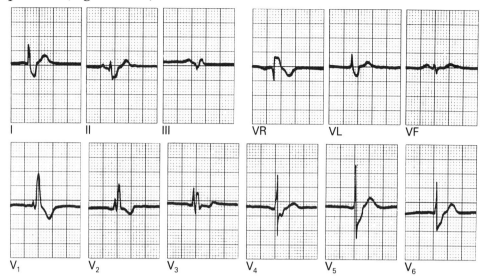

Fig. 7.30 Right bundle branch block

In some cases only one of the fascicles (anterior or posterior) is blocked. This can be detected by analysis of the cardiac axis (see Annex A for details).

If there is a bifascicular block with an acute myocardial infarction, there is a high chance of the patient going into complete (third degree) heart block. Cardiac pacing is therefore recommended. Alternatively, in the absence of an acute infarction, prophylactic pacing is not required with bifascicular block.

If the bundle branch block is associated with a prolonged PR interval (i.e. first degree heart block), then there is a risk of the patient progressing to complete heart block because the remaining bundle is usually diseased.

9. Is there an idioventricular rhythm (IVR)?

This occurs when the ventricles have taken over as the cardiac pacemaker. In view of their slow intrinsic rate of depolarization the heart rate is usually slow (<40 beats/min).

Acute IVR usually occurs after a myocardial infarction. In these cases the IVR occurs in runs, interspersed with a normal sinus rhythm. The ventricular rate is commonly 60–120 beats/min. Treatment is rarely required because the patient is usually haemodynamically stable.

10. Is there ventricular tachycardia?

This occurs when there are three or more consecutive ectopic beats, with a rate greater than 120 beats/min. It is said to be sustained if it lasts more than 30 s (Figure 7.31).

**Fig. 7.31
Ventricular
tachycardia**

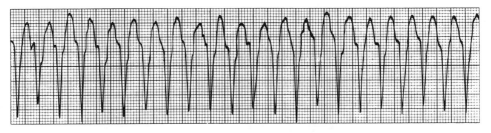

Ventricular tachycardia produces an almost regular rhythm with a wide QRS complex. The rate usually varies between 140 and 250 beats/min.

A regular, broad QRS complex tachycardia can also be due to a supraventricular rhythm with an aberrant conduction. These two dysrhythmias **must be distinguished because pharmacological treatment following a misdiagnosis can be fatal**. After myocardial infarction it is always safer to assume a ventricular origin for this type of tachycardia. Other distinguishing features are listed in Table 7.1.

Table 7.1 Ventricular tachycardia compared with SVT with aberrant conduction

	VT	SVT + aberrant conduction
Fusion beats	Yes	No
Capture beats	Yes	No
Axis change	Yes	No
Concordance	Yes	No
Q in V6	Lost	Present
P waves	Absent or not connected with the QRS	Precede QRS

Fusion beats are produced when the atrial electrical impulse partially depolarizes the ventricular muscle, which has not been fully depolarized by the ventricular ectopic.

Capture beats occur when the atrial electrical impulse completely depolarizes the ventricle before it is depolarized by the ventricular ectopic. The effect is a normal QRS complex in the midst of the ventricular ectopics.

Axis alteration during ventricular tachycardia can only be determined if both the current and previous 12-lead ECG are available. All the limb leads will need to be monitored so that the axis can be plotted accurately (see Annex A).

Concordance occurs when all the V leads have the same shape and direction. Consequently, a 12-lead ECG is required.

If the QRS complex was broad before the tachycardia started and the shape did not change after the tachycardia commenced, then the dysrhythmia is likely to be a SVT with aberrant conduction.

Torsades de Pointes is a type of ventricular tachycardia where the cardiac axis is constantly changing in a regular fashion (see Figure 7.32).

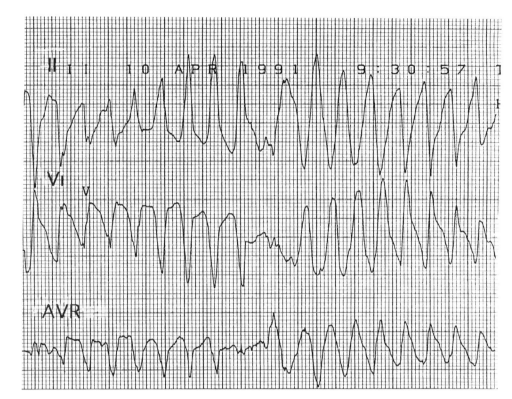

Fig. 7.32 Torsades de Pointes, showing axis change

It looks like the twisting of a helix on the rhythm strip because the amplitude of the QRS complex varies with time. It can be idiosyncratic or due to class 1a anti-arrhythmic agents which increase the QT interval (normally 0.35–0.42 s). This condition can end spontaneously or degenerate into VF.

Ventricular flutter is a further type of broad complex tachycardia. It appears as a sine wave, in which it is difficult to identify the P, QRS and T waves. However, these broad complexes can be distinguished from VF, because they are consistent in size. This condition is associated with a profound fall in the cardiac output.

7.6 SUMMARY

Always treat the patient: not the rhythm.

Is there any electrical activity?

No: asystole
Yes: not asystole

Are there recognizable complexes?

No: ventricular fibrillation
Yes: not ventricular fibrillation

What is the ventricular rate?

What is the rhythm?

P waves:

Are there any abnormal P waves?

Shape?
Timing: earlier or later than normal?

Is there atrial flutter?

Are there the same number of P waves as QRS complexes?

Yes: what is the PR interval?
No: is the PR interval constant?
is the RR interval constant?

Is the QRS duration normal?

Yes: normal ventricular conduction
No: abnormal ventricular conduction
Shape?
Timing: earlier or later than normal?
Frequency?
Supraventricular ectopic focus
Bundle branch block
Idioventricular rhythm
Ventricular tachycardia

The cardiac axis

This can swing like a pendulum depending on the position of the heart in the chest and, more importantly, the relative amounts of functioning muscle in the right and left sides of the heart. If the axis becomes more horizontal, it is said to be deviating to the left.

This is significant when it is 30° above the horizontal line (−30°). If the axis becomes more vertical, it is said to be deviating to the right. This becomes significant when it passes the vertical (+90°) (Figure 7.33).

Fig. 7.33 The QRS axis

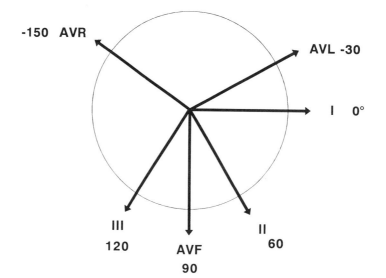

It is simply by convention that the angles above the horizontal line are considered negative, and the ones below, positive.

Two methods will be described to determine the cardiac axis:

METHOD 1: INSPECTING ALL SIX VERTICAL LEADS

1. First determine in which recording lead the QRS is both the smallest and has an equal amount of the complex above and below the baseline. This lead (lead x) is at 90° to the cardiac axis. Using Figure 7.34 as an example, lead x is AVL. Using Figure 7.33, it can be seen that the lead at 90° to this, i.e. the cardiac axis, is either II or −II.
2. To determine which is correct depends on the direction of the impulse along the axis. You will remember that if the electrical impulse moves towards an electrode then there is an upward (positive) deflection. Consequently, if the QRS in II is mainly above the baseline then the impulse is moving towards that lead

position (Figure 7.34). The opposite would apply if the impulse was travelling away from this electrode.

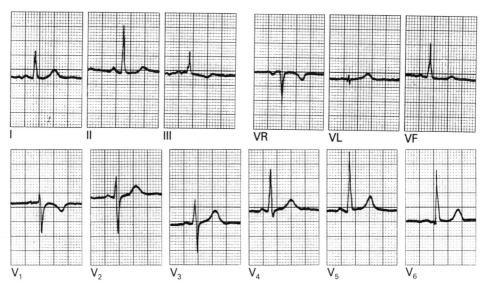

Fig. 7.34 ECG example

Reviewing the trace in Figure 7.34, it can be seen that the majority of the QRS complex in II is above the baseline. Therefore the cardiac axis lies along II.

3. Fine tuning ($\pm 15°$) of the axis determination is achieved by reviewing the relative distribution of the QRS complexes in lead x. If there is slightly more above the baseline, then $+15°$ should be added to the axis assessment derived in the previous paragraph. Conversely, if there is slightly more of the QRS below the baseline, $15°$ is subtracted from the axis assessment.

METHOD 2: INSPECTING LEADS I AND AVF

In this method a vector diagram is constructed.

1. Determine the net deflection in lead I, by subtracting the number of small vertical squares of the R wave deflection from the number of squares of the S or Q wave deflection. The result is plotted along I in Figure 7.34. Using Figure 7.33 again, the R wave is 9.5 small squares and the Q wave 0. This gives a net deflection of 9.5.

2. The same procedure is repeated for lead AVF and the result plotted in Figure 7.35.

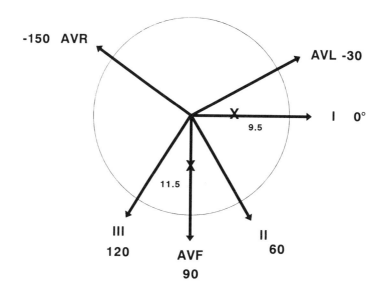

**Fig. 7.35
Marking the
deflections in I
and AVF**

Using the example ECG, this gives a net deflection of 11.5 − 0 = 11.5 small squares. Figure 7.35 shows these two points plotted.

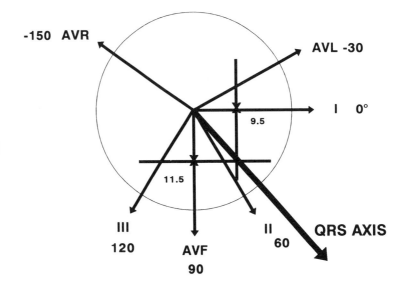

**Fig. 7.36   Plotting
the vector**

3. The resulting intercept of two lines, drawn perpendicularly through these points, will give the axis of the heart (Figure 7.36).

Left axis deviation can follow positional changes in the heart, such as elevation of the diaphragm, or electrical changes associated with left ventricular hypertrophy, left bundle branch block, left anterior fascicular block and right ventricular ectopic rhythms.

Electrical changes associated with right ventricular hypertrophy, right bundle branch block, left posterior fascicular block and left ventricular ectopic rhythms can result in the cardiac axis swinging to the right.

Annex B
Re-entrant tachycardias

WOLFE–PARKINSON–WHITE (WPW) SYNDROME

In this condition, an aberrant pathway bypasses the A-V node, and connects the atrial conducting system directly with the ventricular muscle. Consequently, the atrial impulse can get to the ventricles by two routes. The part of the impulse which goes via the bypass will get to the ventricles quicker than normal as it avoids the resistance in the A-V node. As a result the PR interval is shorter than normal (0.12 s) (Figure 7.37).

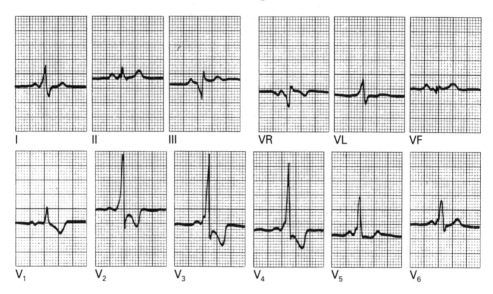

Fig. 7.37
Wolfe–
Parkinson–White
syndrome

As the distal part of this aberrant pathway is not connected with the Bundle of His, ordinary ventricular muscle initially depolarizes.

As this is going on, the rest of the conduction is proceeding normally through the A-V node. Eventually this impulse arrives at the Bundle of His, and the rest of the ventricular depolarization can continue normally. This initial abnormal depolarization is demonstrated, on the ECG, with a slow rise at the beginning of the QRS complex (Figure 7.37). This is known as the delta wave.

LOWN–GANONG–LEVINE (LGL) SYNDROME

This is similar to WPW in that an aberrant conduction pathway bypasses the A-V node. However, this connects with the normal ventricular conducting system, just distal to the A-V node. The effect is to produce a short PR interval (<0.12 s) and a normal, narrow QRS with no delta wave.

Practical skill station
Static dysrhythmia recognition

AIMS

To reinforce practically the knowledge of dysrhythmia recognition gained in theoretical sessions.

To allow candidates to demonstrate proficiency at dysrhythmia recognition using 12-lead ECGs and rhythm strips.

TEACHING TECHNIQUE

A group discussion format is used, in which candidates are asked to demonstrate their knowledge and understanding of the dysrhythmia recognition system taught in the manual and lecture.

TESTING

Candidates are informally assessed on their performance during this skill station. The formal assessment is a written rhythm recognition paper taken on the final day.

Practical skill station
Dynamic dysrhythmia recognition
and defibrillation

AIMS

To reinforce practically the knowledge of dysrhythmia recognition gained in theoretical sessions.

To reinforce the knowledge of treatment protocols gained in theoretical sessions.

To practice a safe and efficient method of defibrillation.

TEACHING TECHNIQUE

Rhythms generated by a computer are displayed on a large screen. The rhythm is identified, and the appropriate treatment protocol revised.

Defibrillation is practised using a defibrillation manikin.

TESTING

Candidates are assessed on their performance during this skill station. Furthermore each candidate must demonstrate a safe and effective technique of defibrillation.

——— 8 ———
Treatment protocols

Objectives

After studying this chapter you should be able to:

- Understand the order of treatments in cardiac arrest rhythms
- Understand the order of treatments in bradyarrhythmias
- Understand the order of treatments in tachyarrhythmias
- Given a simulated patient model, demonstrate the correct application of treatment protocols during resuscitation

---

This chapter deals with the nature and order of electrical and pharmacological treatments for various dysrhythmias. In order to apply the protocols correctly the advanced cardiac life support (ACLS) provider must be proficient at dysrhythmia recognition, and have a thorough knowledge of the defibrillator and of drugs used. These points have been dealt with in earlier chapters.

The protocols are presented as algorithms in three groups:

1. Cardiac arrest rhythms: ventricular fibrillation (VF), asystole, electromechanical dissociation (EMD)
2. Bradyarrhythmias
3. Tachyarrhythmias: ventricular tachycardia (VT), supraventricular tachycardia (SVT), wide complex tachycardia

The Annexes deal with the following practical skills:

Annex A: defibrillation
Annex B: central venous cannulation
Annex C: needle thoracocentesis
Annex D: chest drain insertion
Annex E: pericardiocentesis

Paediatric treatment protocols are shown in Chapter 9.

Remember: treat the patient not the monitor.

8.1 VENTRICULAR FIBRILLATION

The adult ventricular fibrillation algorithm is shown in Figure 8.1.

Fig. 8.1 The ventricular fibrillation algorithm

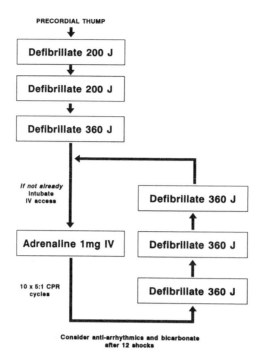

Do not interrupt cardiopulmonary resuscitation (CPR) for more than 10 s except for defibrillation.

8.2 ASYSTOLE

The adult asystole algorithm is shown in Figure 8.2.

Fig. 8.2 The algorithm for asystole

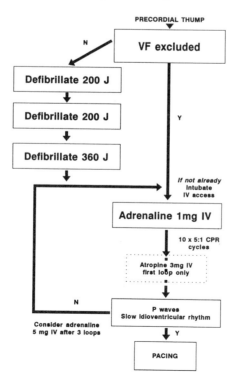

Do not interrupt CPR for more than 10 s except for defibrillation.

8.3 ELECTROMECHANICAL DISSOCIATION

The adult EMD protocol is shown in Figure 8.3.

Fig. 8.3 The algorithm for electro-mechanical dissociation

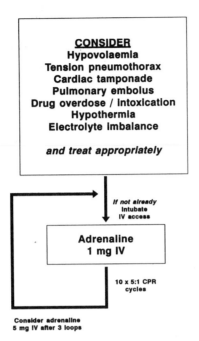

The outcome from primary EMD is poor. However if a secondary cause for EMD exists and this is found and treated promptly the outlook dramatically improves. Thus the main aim in treating a patient in EMD is to assess rapidly whether a treatable cause exists, and to treat it promptly and effectively. Treatable causes fall into two main groups: mechanical abnormalities (treated by correcting the mechanical problem) and biochemical abnormalities (treated with calcium chloride).

8.3.1 Mechanical abnormalities

These causes of secondary EMD have potentially the best outlook (with the exception of massive pulmonary embolus). In general the heart, in the early stages at least, is still able to pump, but is prevented from doing so because of either inadequate filling or constriction.

8.3.1.1 Hypovolaemia

Hypovolaemia of such a degree that it causes EMD is usually due to bleeding. Trauma with its attendant problems is a common cause in all age groups; other causes include ruptured aortic aneurysm and massive gastrointestinal bleeding. Hypovolaemia should always be considered in children: this is dealt with in Chapter 9.

Treatment consists of rapid replacement of the intravascular volume with appropriate fluids, coupled with treatment of the underlying cause.

External cardiac massage is less effective in the hypovolaemic patient, and, if suitably skilled help is available, thoracotomy and internal cardiac massage should be considered. It must be emphasized that thoracotomy is only a temporizing measure, and should only be performed if immediate treatment of the underlying cause of hypovolaemia can be undertaken.

8.3.1.2 Tension pneumothorax

This may be either the primary cause of the arrest or secondary to therapeutic manoeuvres (especially central venous line placement) during the treatment of VF or asystole. The diagnosis is clinical and is made by searching for the following signs:

Unilateral absence of breath sounds
Tracheal deviation

Once the diagnosis has been made the chest should be decompressed rapidly, initially by needle thoracocentesis (Annex C), and then by chest drain placement (Annex D).

Time should not be wasted taking a chest X-ray if this diagnosis is suspected.

8.3.1.3 Pericardial tamponade

This is a difficult diagnosis during cardiac arrest, and a high index of suspicion is necessary if it is to be made. The history may occasionally be diagnostic (for instance stabbing over the precordium); examination is rarely helpful as all the signs of Beck's triad (venous pressure elevation, muffled heart sounds, and decline in arterial pressure) are obscured by the arrest itself. Thus, if other treatable causes of EMD have been eliminated, and a satisfactory output cannot be obtained with external cardiac massage, needle pericardiocentesis should be performed (Annex E).

8.3.1.4 Pulmonary embolus

This diagnosis can only be made on the history. There is no simple treatment, but it is said that vigorous external cardiac massage may occasionally dislodge the clot. In centres that have the facilities, immediate cardiopulmonary bypass followed by operative removal of the clot is life-saving.

8.3.2 Electrolyte imbalance

The use of calcium chloride in EMD has been restricted to the specific indications shown in the algorithm.

Hyperkalaemia and hypocalcaemia may be known to exist from previous tests, but are frequently only discovered biochemically after the resuscitation has failed. More often biochemical abnormality can be predicted from the history. For instance a patient in end-stage renal disease who is dependent on haemodialysis is likely to be hyperkalaemic, and a patient suffering from hydrofluoric acid burns is likely to be hypocalcaemic.

Many patients with ischaemic heart disease are on calcium antagonists, and this information should be actively sought during the resuscitation.

ECG changes may occasionally be diagnostic. These ECG changes are shown in Table 8.1.

Table 8.1   ECG changes

	Hyperkalaemia	Hypocalcaemia
P	Flattened	Normal
QRS	Widened	Normal
QT	Normal	Prolonged
T	Peaked	Normal

8.3.3 Other conditions

Hypothermia and drug overdose are covered in chapter 10.

8.4 BRADYCARDIAS

A bradycardia is defined as a ventricular rate of less than 60. When deciding whether to treat a bradycardia two questions need to be answered: first, 'Does the patient exhibit symptoms and signs that need treatment?' and second, 'Does the rhythm have the potential to cause cardiac standstill?'

Significant symptoms and signs are:

Chest pain
Dyspnoea
Hypotension (systolic <90 mmHg)
Congestive cardiac failure
Altered mental status

If any of these are present then the bradycardia should be treated.

The adult bradycardia algorithm is shown in Figure 8.4.

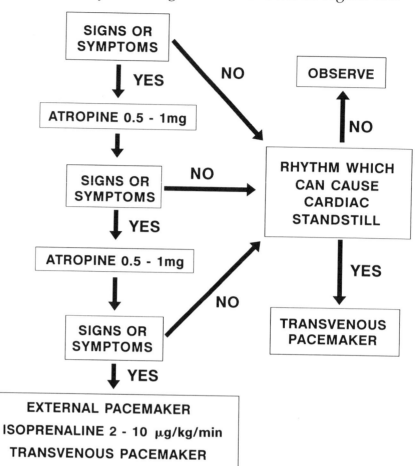

Fig. 8.4
Algorithm
for the
management of
bradycardias

The recognition of dysrhythmias was dealt with in Chapter 7. Two bradycardiac rhythms have the potential to cause cardiac standstill, particularly after myocardial infarction. These are:

Second degree block: Mobitz type II
Third degree block

If these are present then a demand pacemaker is required.

8.5 VENTRICULAR TACHYCARDIA

Patients who have VT may be in a number of clinical states. The immediate treatment of the dysrhythmia is governed by their clinical condition rather than by the dysrhythmia itself. In other words:

Remember: treat the patient not the monitor.

The first part of the VT algorithm is shown in Figure 8.5:

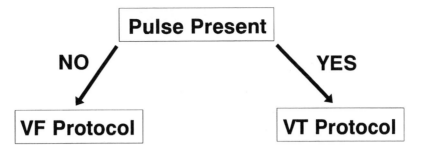

Fig. 8.5 Management of pulseless ventricular tachycardia

The VF algorithm was shown in Figure 8.1, and the second part of the VT algorithm is shown in Figure 8.6.

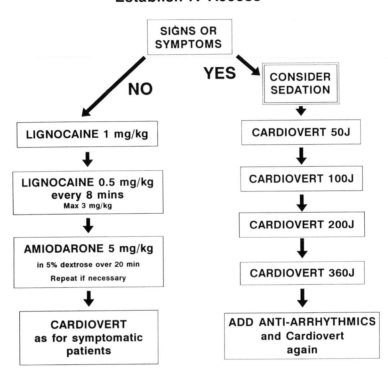

Fig. 8.6 The adult ventricular tachycardia algorithm

Significant symptoms and signs are:

Chest pain
Dyspnoea
Hypotension (systolic <90 mmHg)
Congestive cardiac failure
Altered mental status

Synchronous cardioversion is theoretically safer in VT, since DC countershock at the wrong part of the cardiac cycle can precipitate VF. However if the patient is symptomatic (see above) the delays that frequently occur while waiting for synchronization may be counterproductive, and unsynchronized cardioversion is advised. Furthermore if the VT is very fast the QRS and T waves can be difficult to distinguish, and unsynchronized cardioversion may be safer. In the asymptomatic patient who requires elective cardioversion, a synchronized shock is recommended.

8.6 SUPRAVENTRICULAR TACHYCARDIA

The adult SVT algorithm is shown in Figure 8.7.

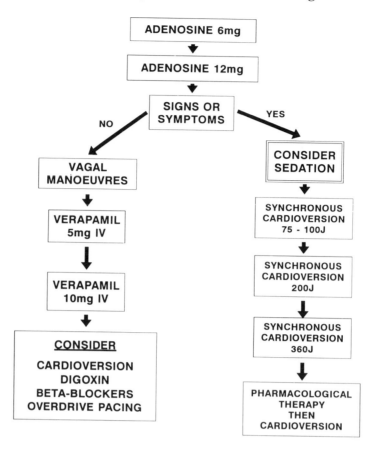

Fig. 8.7 The adult supraventricular tachycardia algorithm

Remember: treat the patient not the monitor

Significant symptoms and signs are:

Chest pain
Dyspnoea
Hypotension (systolic <90 mmHg)
Congestive cardiac failure
Altered mental status

8.7 WIDE COMPLEX TACHYCARDIA

Occasionally it can be difficult to distinguish between ventricular tachycardia and supraventricular tachycardia with aberrant conduction. If the patient is symptomatic it is more important to treat than to diagnose. The safest course is to treat wide complex tachycardia as though it were ventricular in origin. Figure 8.8 shows the algorithm for undiagnosed wide complex tachycardia.

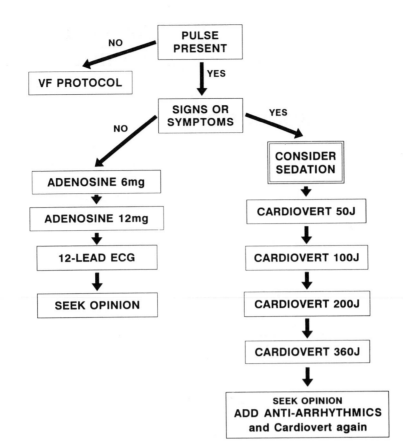

Fig. 8.8
Management of
wide complex
tachycardias

Remember: treat the patient not the monitor

INTRODUCTION

Defibrillation is the single most efficacious treatment of cardiac arrest in adults. In order to achieve the optimum outcome, defibrillation must be performed quickly and efficiently. This requires:

Correct paddle selection
Correct paddle placement
Good paddle contact
Correct energy selection

Many defibrillators are available. ACLS providers should make sure they are familiar with those they may have to use.

Correct paddle selection

Most defibrillators are supplied with adult paddles (13 cm diameter, or equivalent area). For infants, 4.5 cm diameter paddles are used, and for children 8 cm diameter paddles.

Correct paddle placement

The usual placement is antero-lateral. One paddle is put over the apex in the mid-axillary line, and the other is just to the right of the sternum, immediately below the clavicle (Figure 8.9).

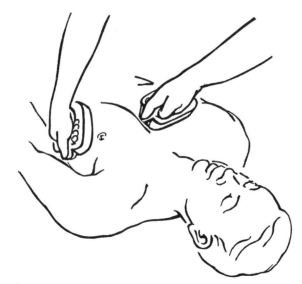

**Fig. 8.9
Standard antero-lateral paddle placement**

If the anterior-posterior placement is used, one paddle is placed just to the left side of the lower part of the sternum, and the other just below the tip of the left scapula (Figure 8.10).

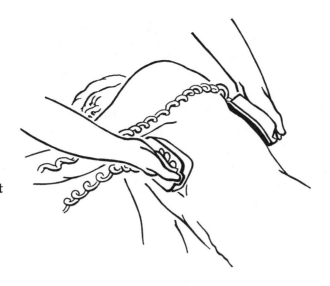

**Fig. 8.10
Antero-posterior
paddle placement**

Good paddle contact

Gel pads or electrode gel should always be used (if the latter is used, care should be taken not to join the two areas of application). Firm pressure should be applied to the paddles.

Correct energy selection

The recommended levels are shown in the relevant (adult and paediatric) VF protocols.

SAFETY

A defibrillator delivers enough current to **cause** cardiac arrest. The user must ensure that other rescuers are not in physical contact with the patient (or the trolley) at the moment the shock is delivered.

PROCEDURE

1. Apply gel pads or electrode gel.
2. Select the correct paddles.
3. Select the energy required.
4. Press the charge button.
5. Wait until the defibrillator is charged.
6. Place the electrodes onto the pads of gel, and apply firm pressure.
7. Shout "Stand back!"
8. Check that all other rescuers are clear.
9. Deliver the shock.

Basic life support should be interrupted for the shortest possible time (points 6–9).

Annex B
Central venous cannulation

Cannulation of peripheral veins is not recommended following a cardiac arrest because the procedure can be time consuming and the drug transit time from the periphery to the heart is prolonged. Therefore, catheterization of a central vein is recommended and, paradoxically, relatively easy to perform. However, in the circumstances of a cardiac arrest, it may be necessary for someone to catheterize a central vein safely and quickly but without the benefit of a great deal of experience. Therefore, a technique is required which is easy to perform and has a high success rate with few complications. Many approaches and different types of equipment have been described to secure central venous access. This annex describes two approaches (internal jugular and subclavian), using a single technique which can be used for either. The techniques described are the ones found to be successful in both experienced and inexperienced hands. No further justification of their choice is offered. For those already skilled at central venous cannulation using a different technique (with an acceptable rate of complications), carry on!

THE SELDINGER TECHNIQUE

Although initially described for use with arterial cannulation, this technique is very suitable for central venous cannulation and is associated with an increased success rate. It relies on the insertion of a guide wire into the vein over which a suitable catheter is passed. As a relatively small needle is used to introduce the wire, damage to adjacent structures is reduced.

The course of the central veins is demonstrated in Figure 8.11.

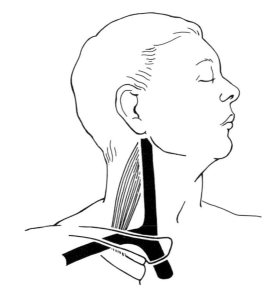

Fig. 8.11 The course of the central veins of the neck

Having decided which approach to use (see below), the skin must be prepared and towelled. Full aseptic precautions are necessary as a 'no-touch' technique is not possible. The equipment to be used is then checked and prepared. In particular, the floppy end of the wire is identified and free passage of the guide wire through the needle is ascertained. The needle is then attached to a syringe and percutaneous venepuncture made. Once the vein is identified by aspiration of blood, the syringe is removed taking care to avoid the entry of air (usually by placing a thumb over the end of the needle). The floppy end of the guide wire is then inserted into the needle and advanced 4–5 cm into the vein. The needle is then removed over the wire, taking care not to remove the wire with the needle. The catheter is then loaded on to the wire, ensuring that the proximal end of the wire protrudes from the catheter. While holding on to the proximal end of the wire, the catheter and wire are inserted into the vein. The wire is then removed, holding the catheter in position. A syringe can now be reattached and blood aspirated to confirm placement of the catheter in the vein. If difficulty is encountered inserting the wire, the needle and wire must be removed together. Failure to do this may result in the tip of the wire being damaged as it is withdrawn past the needle point, thereby making withdrawal difficult. After 3 min gentle pressure to reduce bleeding, the needle can be reintroduced. Occasionally it may be necessary to make a small incision in the skin to facilitate passage of the catheter.

APPROACH TO THE CENTRAL VEINS

Whenever possible the patient should be placed in a head-down position to dilate the vein and reduce the risk of air embolus.

The subclavian vein: infraclavicular approach

1. The patient is placed supine, with arms at the side and head turned away from the side of the puncture. Occasionally it may be advantageous to place a small support (a 500 ml bag of fluid!) under the scapula of the side of approach, to raise the clavicle above the shoulder.
2. Standing on the same side as that to be punctured (usually the right), the operator should identify the midclavicular point and the suprasternal notch.
3. Under sterile conditions the needle is inserted 1 cm below the midclavicular point and advanced posterior to the clavicle towards a finger in the suprasternal notch. The syringe and needle should be kept horizontal during advancement, aspirating at all times.
4. Entry into the vein is confirmed by blood entering the syringe.

The catheter is then introduced via a guide wire as already described.

5. A chest X-ray should be taken as soon as possible to exclude a pneumothorax and confirm correct positioning of the catheter.

Complications:

1. **Pneumothorax**: the dome of the pleura lies above the level of the clavicle and is easily punctured if the needle is advanced at too deep an angle. Hence bilateral attempts are not recommended.
2. **Haemothorax**: usually from puncture of the subclavian artery or more rarely tearing of the vein.
3. **Brachial plexus injury**: wrong direction of insertion of needle.
4. **Tracheal puncture**: needle inserted too far.
5. **Infection**: usually at site of entry, due to poor aseptic technique.

The main advantage of using the subclavian vein is that it is prevented from collapsing by the surrounding tissues and therefore is more easily identified in shocked patients. However, there are many potential complications of this route and its use is being challenged by the internal jugular vein because of its apparent safety.

The internal jugular vein: para-carotid approach

This method is based on the fact that the internal jugular vein runs parallel to the carotid artery in the carotid sheath and therefore rotation of the head, obesity and individual variations in anatomy have less effect on the location of the vein.

1. The patient is placed supine with the arms at the side and the head in a neutral position.
2. An attempt should be made to try to detect the carotid pulse by standing at the head of the patient, identifying the thyroid cartilage and palpating with the fingers of the left hand, perpendicular to the coronal plane (the right internal jugular being the one most commonly used initially).
3. Under sterile conditions, with the fingers of the left hand 'guarding' the carotid artery, a needle is inserted 0.5 cm lateral to the artery.
4. The needle is slowly advanced caudally, parallel to the sagittal plane at an angle of 45° to the skin, aspirating at all times.
5. Entry into the vein is confirmed by blood entering the syringe. The catheter is then introduced via a guide wire as already described.
6. If the vein is not entered at the first attempt, then subsequent punctures should be directed slightly more laterally (never doubling back towards the artery).

Although a chest X-ray should be taken it is less urgent than when using the subclavian vein, as the catheter is more likely to be correctly positioned and the incidence of pneumothorax is much lower with this approach.

Complications:

1. **Failure**: usually because the initial attempt is made too far laterally.
2. **Haematoma**: due to puncture of the carotid artery. Fortunately this is less of a problem with this method as pressure can be applied to the artery to minimize bleeding.
3. **Pneumothorax**: rare, as the attempt is made well above the pleura (unless too long a needle is used!).
4. **Puncture of vertebral vessels, oesophagus, trachea**: rare, as these structures are medial to the carotid artery.

Annex C
Needle thoracocentesis

MINIMUM EQUIPMENT

Alcohol swabs
Large needle with IV cannula (16 g or more)
20 ml syringe

PROCEDURE

1. Identify the second intercostal space in the midclavicular line on the side of the pneumothorax (the **opposite** side to the direction of tracheal deviation).
2. Swab the chest wall with surgical prep or an alcohol swab.
3. Attach the syringe to the cannula.
4. Insert the cannula into the chest wall, just above the rib below, aspirating all the time.
5. If air is aspirated remove the needle, leaving the plastic cannula in place.
6. Tape the cannula in place and proceed to chest drain insertion (see Annex D) as soon as possible.

If needle thoracocentesis is attempted, and the patient does not have a tension pneumothorax, the chance of causing a pneumothorax is 10%–20%. Patients who have had this procedure must have a chest X-ray, and will require chest drainage if ventilated.

Annex D
Chest drain placement

MINIMUM EQUIPMENT

Skin prep and surgical drapes
Scalpel
Large clamps × 2
Suture
(Local anaesthetic)
Scissors
Chest drain tube

PROCEDURE

1. Decide on the insertion site (usually the fifth intercostal space in the mid-axillary line) on the side with the pneumothorax.
2. Swab the chest wall with surgical prep or an alcohol swab.
3. Use local anaesthetic if necessary.
4. Make a 2–3 cm skin incision along the line of the intercostal space, just above the rib below.
5. Bluntly dissect through the subcutaneous tissues just over the top of the rib below, and puncture the parietal pleura with the tip of the clamp.
6. Put a gloved finger into the incision and clear the path into the pleura.
7. Advance the chest drain tube into the pleural space.
8. Ensure the tube is in the pleural space by listening for air movement, and by looking for fogging of the tube during expiration.
9. Connect the chest drain tube to an underwater seal.
10. Suture the drain in place, and secure with tape.
11. Obtain a chest X-ray.

Annex E
Pericardiocentesis

MINIMUM EQUIPMENT

ECG monitor
(Local anaesthetic)
20 ml syringe
Skin prep and surgical drapes
6 inch over the needle cannula (16 g or 18 g)

PROCEDURE (FIGURES 8.12 AND 8.13)

1. Closely monitor the ECG during the procedure. Look for an acute injury pattern (if not already present due to myocardial infarction) i.e. ST segment changes or widened QRS. These indicate ventricular damage by the needle.

2. Swab the xiphoid and subxiphoid areas with surgical prep or an alcohol swab.

3. Use local anaesthetic if necessary.

4. Assess the patient for any significant mediastinal shift if possible.

5. Attach the syringe to the needle.

6. Puncture the skin 1–2 cm inferior to the left side of the xiphoid junction at a 45° angle.

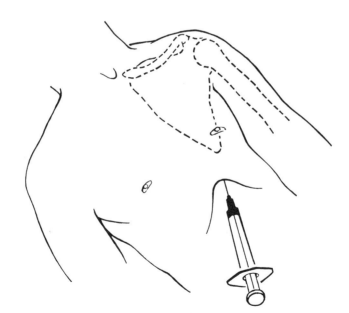

**Fig. 8.12
Needle pericar-
diocentesis –
direction**

7. Advance the needle towards the tip of the left scapula, aspirating all the time.

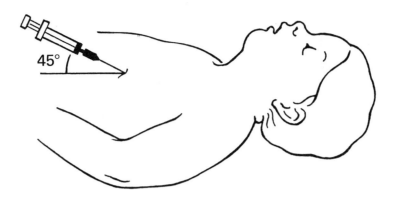

Fig. 8.13
Needle pericar-
diocentesis – angle

45°

8. Watch the ECG monitor for signs of myocardial injury.

9. Once fluid is withdrawn aspirate as much as possible (unless it is possible to withdraw limitless amounts of blood in which case a ventricle has probably been entered).

10. If the procedure is successful, remove the needle, leaving the cannula in the pericardial sac. Secure in place and seal with a three-way tap. This allows later repeat aspirations should tamponade recur.

Practical skill station
Central venous access

AIMS

To reinforce practically the procedure involved in central venous access.
To allow candidates to demonstrate proficiency at central venous access.

TEACHING TECHNIQUE

The procedure will be demonstrated by the instructor using the central venous cannulation trainer and then candidates will be allowed to practice.

TESTING

Candidates are informally assessed on their performance during this skill station. No formal testing is undertaken.

Practical skill station
Intravenous access

AIMS

To reinforce practically the procedure involved in intravenous access.
To allow candidates to demonstrate proficiency at intravenous access.

TEACHING TECHNIQUE

The procedure will be demonstrated by the instructor using the IV trainer and then candidates will be allowed to practice.

TESTING

Candidates are informally assessed on their performance during this skill station. No formal testing is undertaken.

9

Paediatric life support

Objectives

After studying this chapter you should be able to:

- Understand the pathophysiology of cardiac arrest in childhood

- Understand the principles of paediatric basic life support

- Understand the principles of paediatric advanced cardiac life support

- Given a simulated patient model, demonstrate the proficient provision of basic life support to a child

- Demonstrate proficiency at basic and advanced airway control in children

9.1 CAUSES OF CARDIAC ARREST IN CHILDHOOD

Most deaths in infancy and childhood occur in previously well or potentially healthy children. In the newborn period, the commonest causes of death are due either to factors associated with prematurity (e.g. respiratory immaturity, cerebral haemorrhage, or infection due to immaturity of the immune response), or to congenital abnormalities.

In the first year of life the condition we describe as 'cot death' is the commonest cause of death. Some infant victims of this condition have previously unrecognized respiratory or metabolic diseases, while in others no adequate cause for death is found at detailed post-mortem examination. This latter group of children are described as victims of the Sudden Infant Death syndrome. After the age of one, trauma is the commonest cause of death, and remains so until well into early adult life.

Cardiac arrest in infancy and childhood is rarely due to primary cardiac disease. Excluding the Sudden Infant Death syndrome the majority are secondary to hypoxia. This may have resulted from conditions such as birth asphyxia, epiglottitis, inhalation of foreign body, bronchiolitis, asthma or pneumothorax. Whatever the cause, by the time cardiac arrest occurs, the child has had a period of respiratory insufficiency which will have caused respiratory acidosis (from carbon dioxide retention), and metabolic acidosis (from hypoxia). The combination of hypoxia and acidosis causes cell damage and death in sensitive organs such as the brain, liver and kidney, before myocardial damage is severe enough to cause cardiac arrest.

The next major cause of cardiac arrest is circulatory failure (shock). This will have resulted either from blood loss or fluid redistribution from within the circulation. The former is due to trauma, whilst the latter can be the result of gastroenteritis, burns, sepsis, anaphylaxis etc. The end point once again is tissue hypoxia, metabolic acidosis and cardiac arrest. The pathways leading to cardiac arrest in children are summarized in Figure 9.1.

Fig. 9.1 Pathways leading to cardiac arrest in childhood (with examples of underlying causes)

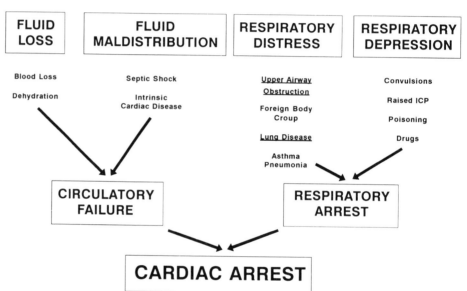

The aetiology of cardiac arrest in children should be contrasted with that in adults, where the primary cause of arrest is often cardiac, and cardiorespiratory function may be near normal until the time that the arrest occurs. In this situation, hypoxia and ischaemic tissue damage occur after the heart has stopped, and may, therefore, be prevented by prompt treatment.

The worst outcome is in children who arrive apnoeic and pulseless at an Accident and Emergency department. These children have a less than 5% chance of intact neurological survival, since there has often been a prolonged period of hypoxia and ischaemia before adequate cardiopulmonary resuscitation (CPR). Earlier recognition of seriously ill children and more widespread paediatric CPR training could improve the outcome.

9.2 RECOGNITION OF RESPIRATORY AND CIRCULATORY FAILURE

As the outcome from cardiac arrest in childhood is so poor, it is vital to recognize the signs of respiratory and/or circulatory failure **whatever their cause** before the arrest occurs.

The following signs are suggestive of respiratory failure:

Tachypnoea
Use of accessory muscles of respiration
Severe chest retraction
Decreased or absent breath sounds
Restlessness and agitation or decreased level of consciousness
Hypotonia
Cyanosis (late and preterminal sign)

The following signs are suggestive of circulatory failure:

Rapid thready pulse
Rapid deep breathing
Agitation or depressed conscious level
Skin pallor and coldness with poor capillary refill
Oliguria
Hypotension (late sign)

9.3 NOTABLE DIFFERENCES BETWEEN CHILDREN AND ADULTS

Children must not simply be regarded as small adults. There are important anatomical and physiological differences.

Anatomical differences:

Relatively large head with prominent occiput
Small mandible
Large, floppy epiglottis, often obscuring the larynx
Cone-shaped larynx, higher (opposite C2), more anterior
Narrowest part of larynx below the vocal cords
Trachea is soft, short and easily compressed
Chest is relatively small compared with the abdomen

Physiological differences:

Heat lost rapidly due to large surface area:weight ratio
Increased oxygen requirement per kg body weight
Increased caloric requirement per kg body weight
Predominantly diaphragmatic breathers
Pulmonary maturity incomplete until 8 years
Small airways close easily causing ventilation/perfusion inequality
Neonates have poor elastic recoil in their airways

9.4 BASIC LIFE SUPPORT IN CHILDREN

9.4.1 Introduction

Paediatric basic life support is not simply a scaled down version of that provided for adults. Although the general principles are the same, specific techniques are required if the optimum support is to be given. Furthermore the exact techniques employed need to be varied according to the size of the child. A somewhat artificial line is generally drawn between infants (less than 1 year old) and small children (less than 8 years old), and that approach is followed here.

By applying the basic techniques described, a single rescuer can support the vital respiratory and circulatory functions of a collapsed child with no equipment.

9.4.2 The SAFE approach

Additional help should be summoned rapidly. Furthermore it is essential that the rescuer does not become a second victim, and that the child is removed from continuing danger as quickly as possible. These considerations should precede the initial airway assessment. They are summarized in Figure 9.2.

Shout for help

Approach with care

Free from danger

Evaluate ABC

Fig. 9.2 The SAFE approach

9.4.3 Are you alright?

As in adults, the initial simple assessment of responsiveness consists of asking the child "Are you alright?", and **gently** shaking them by the shoulders. Infants and very small children who cannot yet talk, and older children who are very scared are unlikely to reply meaningfully, but may make some sound or open their eyes to the rescuer's voice.

In cases associated with trauma the neck and spine should be immobilized during this manoeuvre. This is achieved by placing one hand firmly on the forehead, while one of the child's arms is shaken gently.

9.4.4 Assessment and treatment

Once the child has been approached correctly and a simple test for unresponsiveness has been carried out, assessment and treatment follow the familiar ABC pattern. The overall sequence of basic life support in cardio-pulmonary arrest is summarized in Figure 9.3.

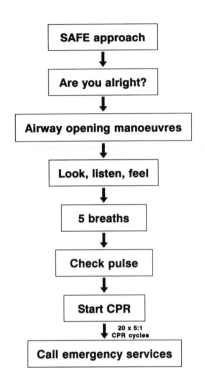

**Fig. 9.3
Sequence of BLS
in paediatric
cardio-pulmonary
arrest**

9.4.4.1 Airway

An obstructed airway may be the primary problem, and correction of the obstruction can result in recovery without further intervention.

If a child is having difficulty breathing, but is conscious, then transport to hospital should be arranged as quickly as possible. A child will often find the best position to maintain their own airway, and should not be forced to adopt a position which they find less comfortable. Attempts to improve a partially maintained airway in an environment where immediate advanced support is not available can be dangerous, since total obstruction may occur.

If the child is not conscious then the patency of the airway should be assessed.

If the child is not breathing it may be because the airway has been blocked by the tongue falling back to obstruct the pharynx. An attempt to open the airway should be made using head tilt/chin lift. The rescuer places the hand nearest to the child's head on the forehead, and applies pressure to tilt the head back gently. The desirable degrees of tilt are: infant, neutral; child, sniffing.

The fingers of the other hand should then be placed under the chin and the chin should be lifted upwards. Care should be taken not to injure the soft tissue of the chin by gripping too hard. Since this action can close the child's mouth, it may be necessary to use the thumb of the same hand to part the lips slightly. The optimal position for airway opening in infants is shown in Figure 9.4.

Fig. 9.4 Airway opening in infants

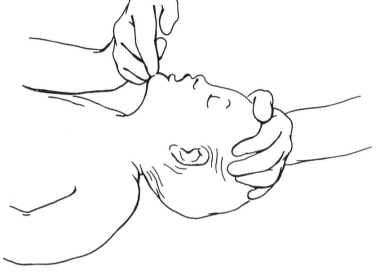

Once this manoeuvre has been carried out the airway should be reassessed using the look, listen, feel technique.

The rescuer places their face above the child's, with the ear over the nose, the cheek over the mouth, and the eyes looking along the line of the chest.

An alternative to the head tilt/chin lift is the jaw thrust. This is achieved by placing two or three fingers under the angle of the mandible bilaterally, and lifting the jaw upwards. This technique may be easier if the rescuer's elbows are resting on the same surface as the child is lying on. A small degree of head tilt may also be applied.

As before, the success or failure of the intervention is assessed using the look, listen, feel technique described above.

It should be noted that if there is a history of trauma then the head tilt/chin lift manoeuvre may exacerbate cervical spine injury. The safest airway intervention in these circumstances is jaw thrust without head tilt. Proper cervical spine control can only be achieved in such cases by a second rescuer maintaining in-line cervical stabilization throughout.

The finger sweep technique often recommended in adults should not be used in children. The child's soft palate is easily damaged and bleeding from within the mouth can worsen the situation. Furthermore foreign bodies may be forced further down the airway; since the child's larynx is cone-shaped, these can get lodged below the cords and become even more difficult to remove.

If a foreign body is not obvious, inspection should be done under direct vision in hospital, and, if appropriate, removal should be attempted using Magills forceps.

9.4.4.2 Breathing

If the airway opening techniques described above do not result in the resumption of breathing, exhaled air resuscitation should be commenced.

While the airway is kept open as described above, the rescuer breathes in and seals their mouth around the victim's mouth, or mouth and nose. If the mouth alone is used then the nose should be pinched closed using the thumb and index fingers of the hand that is maintaining head tilt. Slow exhalation (1–1½ s) by the rescuer should result in the victim's chest rising.

Since children vary in size only general guidance can be given regarding the volume and pressure of inflation, as follows:

The chest should be seen to rise
Inflation pressure may be higher since airways are small
Slow breaths at the lowest pressure reduce gastric distention

If the chest does not rise then the airway is not clear. The usual cause is failure to apply correctly the airway opening techniques discussed above. Thus the first thing to do is to readjust the head tilt/chin lift position, and try again. If this does not work jaw thrust should be tried; it is quite possible for a single rescuer to open the airway using this technique and perform exhaled air resuscitation. However, if two rescuers are present one should maintain the airway while the other breathes for the child. Failure of both head tilt/chin and jaw thrust should lead to the suspicion that a foreign body is causing the obstruction, and the appropriate action should be taken.

Five initial rescue breaths should be given.

9.4.4.3 Circulation

The absence of an adequate circulation is recognized by the absence of a large pulse for 5 s. In small children, as in adults, the carotid artery in the neck can be palpated.

In infants the neck is generally short and fat, and the carotid artery may be difficult to identify. Therefore the brachial artery in the medial aspect of the antecubital fossa or the femoral artery in the groin should be felt (Figure 9.5).

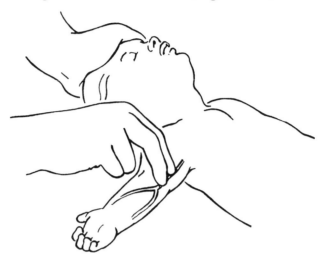

**Fig. 9.5
Feeling for the
brachial pulse**

If the pulse is absent or inadequate (less than 60 beats/min) for 5 s then cardiac compression is required. If the pulse is present and at an adequate rate (over 60 beats/min) but apnoea persists, exhaled air resuscitation must be continued until spontaneous breathing resumes.

The precordial thump is not recommended in children.

9.4.4.4 Cardiac compression

For the best output the child must be placed lying flat on their back, on a hard surface. In infants it is said that the palm of the rescuer's hand can be used for this purpose, but this may prove difficult in practice.

Children vary in size, and the exact nature of the compressions given should reflect this. In general infants (less than 1 year) require a different technique from small children. In children over 8 years of age the method used in adults can be applied with appropriate modifications for their size.

Infants. Since the infant heart is lower with relation to external landmarks when compared with older children and adults, the area of compression is found by imagining a line between the nipples and compressing over the sternum one finger breadth below this line. Two fingers are used to compress the chest to a depth of approximately 1.5–2.5 cm. This is shown in Figure 9.6.

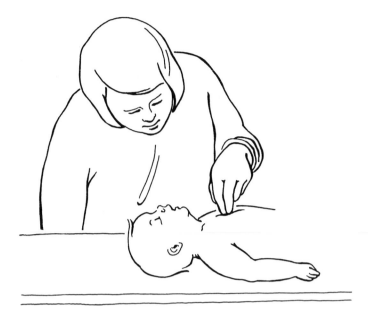

Fig. 9.6 Chest compressions in an infant

Alternatively, infant cardiac compression can be achieved using the hand encircling technique. The infant is held with both the rescuer's hands encircling the chest. The thumbs are placed over the correct part of the sternum (see above) and compression carried out.

Small children. The area of compression is one finger breadth above the xiphisternum. The heel of one hand is used to compress the sternum to a depth of approximately 2.5–3.5 cm (Figure 9.7)

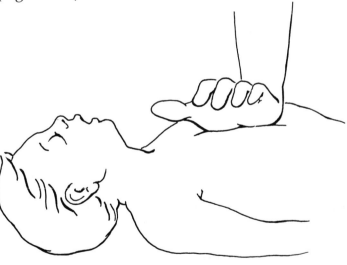

Fig. 9.7 Chest compressions in small children

Larger children. The area of compression is two finger breadths above the xiphisternum. The heels of both hands are used to compress the sternum to a depth of approximately 3–4.5 cm, depending on the size of the child. This is illustrated in Figure 9.8.

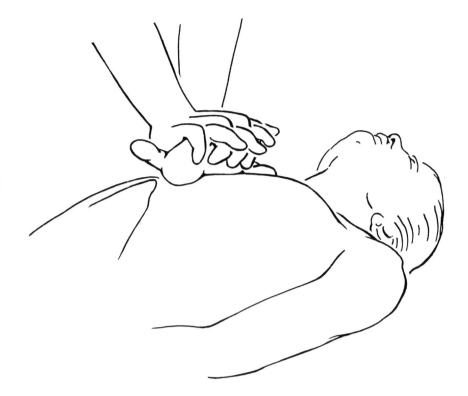

Fig. 9.8 Chest compressions in older children

Once the correct technique has been chosen and the area for compression identified, **five compressions should be given.**

9.4.4.5 Continuing cardiopulmonary resuscitation

A ratio of 5 compressions to 1 ventilation is maintained whatever the number of rescuers. Since the normal heart rate in infants and children is higher than in adults, the optimal compression rate is higher. Infants should receive 20–24 complete cycles per minute (100–120 compressions), small children 16–20 (80–100 compressions), and larger children 14–20 (70–100 compressions) depending on size.

Basic life support must not be interrupted.

In infants, with their requirement for high cycle rates, any time spent readjusting the airway or re-establishing the correct position for compressions will seriously decrease the number of cycles given per minute. This can be a very real problem for the solo rescuer and there is no easy solution. However, slower rates done efficiently are preferred.

The CPR manoeuvres recommended for infants and children are summarized in Table 9.1.

Table 9.1 Summary of BLS techniques in infants and children

	Infant	Small child	Larger child
Airway: head tilt position	Neutral	Sniffing	Sniffing
Breathing: initial slow breaths	2	2	2
Circulation: Pulse check	Brachial or femoral	Carotid	Carotid
Landmark	1 finger breadth below nipple line	1 finger breadth above xiphisternum	2 finger breadths above xiphisternum
Technique	2 fingers or encircling	1 hand	2 hands
Depth	1.5–2.5 cm	2.5–3.5 cm	3–4.5 cm
CPR: ratio	5:1	5:1	5:1
Cycles per min	20–24	16–20	14–20

9.4.5 The choking child

9.4.5.1 Introduction

The vast majority of deaths from foreign body aspiration occur in pre-school children. Virtually anything may be inhaled. The diagnosis is very rarely clear-cut, but should be suspected if the onset of respiratory compromise is sudden and is associated with coughing, gagging and stridor. Airway obstruction may also occur with infections such as acute epiglottitis and croup. In such cases attempts to relieve the obstruction using the methods described below are dangerous. Children with known or suspected infectious causes of obstruction, and those who are still breathing and in whom the cause of obstruction is unclear, should be taken to hospital urgently.

The physical methods of clearing the airway that are described below should therefore only be performed if:

1. The diagnosis of foreign body aspiration is clear-cut, and dyspnoea is increasing or apnoea has occurred.
2. Head tilt/chin lift and jaw thrust have failed to open the airway of an apnoeic child.

131

9.4.5.2 Infants

There is concern that abdominal thrusts may cause intra-abdominal injury in infants. Therefore a combination of back blows and chest thrusts are recommended for the relief of foreign body obstruction in this age group.

The baby is placed along one of the rescuer's arms in a head down position. The rescuer then rests their arm along their thigh, and delivers four back blows with the heel of their free hand (Figure 9.9).

Fig. 9.9 Back blows

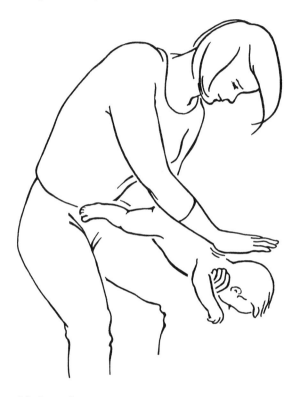

If the obstruction is not relieved the baby is turned over and laid along the rescuer's thigh, still in a head down position. Four chest thrusts are given, using the same landmarks as for cardiac compression but a slower rate.

If an infant is too large to allow the single arm technique to be used, then the same manoeuvres can be performed by lying the baby across the rescuer's lap.

9.4.5.3 Children

In the older child the Heimlich manoeuvre can be used. As in the adult this can be performed with the victim either standing, sitting, kneeling or lying.

If this is to be attempted with the child standing, kneeling or sitting, the rescuer moves behind the victim and passes their arms around them. Due to the height of children it may be necessary for an adult to stand the child on a box or other convenient object to carry out the standing manoeuvre effectively. One hand is formed into a fist and placed against the child's abdomen above the umbilicus and below the xiphisternum. The other hand is placed over the fist, and both hands are thrust sharply upwards into the abdomen. This is repeated ten times unless the object causing the obstruction is expelled before then.

To carry out the Heimlich manoeuvre in a supine child, the rescuer kneels at their feet. If the child is large it may be necessary to kneel astride them. The heel of one hand is placed against the child's abdomen above the umbilicus and below the xiphisternum. The other hand is placed above the first, and both hands are thrust sharply upwards into the abdomen with care being taken to direct the thrust in the midline. This is repeated ten times unless the object causing the obstruction is expelled before then.

9.4.5.4 Putting it all together: Managing a choking child

The sequence of actions necessary to manage a choking child is shown in Figure 9.10.

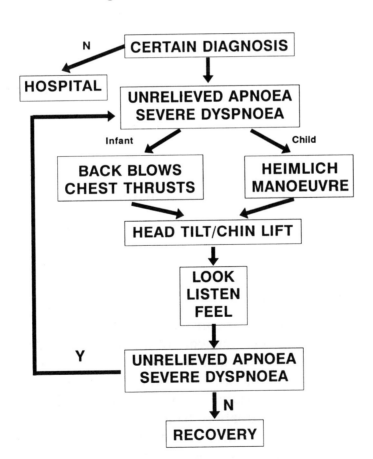

Fig. 9.10
Algorithm for
managing a
choking child

9.5 ADVANCED SUPPORT OF THE AIRWAY AND VENTILATION

Airway and breathing have priority in the resuscitation of patients of all ages, but the rate at which respiratory function can deteriorate in children is particularly rapid. If basic life support techniques fail, it is vital that advanced techniques of obtaining a patent airway, and achieving adequate ventilation and oxygenation, are applied quickly and effectively.

9.5.1 Airway adjuncts

An oropharyngeal (Guedel) airway may be used to try to improve or provide a patent airway in the obtunded patient. The oropharyngeal airway comes in a variety of sizes, from 000 for neonates to size 1 for children (sizes 2–4 for adults). An estimate of the correct size can be made by comparing the airway with the distance from the angle of the child's mouth to the ear lobe. Too small an airway will press against the tongue, while one that is too large will cause trauma.

In the older child the airway can be inserted 'upside down' as in adults. However in babies and young children there is a danger that the soft palate may be damaged using this technique, and it is better to insert the airway the correct way up, under direct vision and using a tongue depressor (a laryngoscope blade will suffice). Despite taking care, an oropharyngeal airway may occasionally cause trauma and bleeding or laryngospasm and vomiting if the gag reflex is present. After inserting an airway the patient should be assessed using look, listen and feel.

Nasopharyngeal airways are not widely used in children. This is partly because small sizes suitable for children are not made and therefore a tracheal tube of appropriate diameter has to be cut to length. Furthermore the vascular nasal mucosa and large adenoids are easily damaged during insertion and may bleed into the airway.

9.5.2 Tracheal intubation

In the deeply unconscious child, the best method of securing the airway is by tracheal intubation. This will facilitate ventilation and protect against the risk of aspiration of regurgitated gastric contents or blood. The oral rather than nasal route is preferred for the reasons stated above. A variety of equipment is needed to facilitate intubation (see Annex A). It is essential that this is checked regularly, to ensure availability and function. A final check should be made immediately prior to intubation.

9.5.2.1 Technique

Preoxygenation. Whenever possible intubation should be preceded by a period of ventilation with 100% oxygen using a bag–valve–mask device.

Infants under 6 months. These children are often best positioned flat without a pillow and the head in neutral. Sometimes a small folded towel placed under the shoulders facilitates extension of the infant head to the neutral position.

A straight-bladed laryngoscope, held in the left hand, is then introduced into the mouth along the right side of the tongue. The aim is to 'pick-up' the epiglottis by passing posterior to it. The laryngoscope is then gently lifted to reveal the vocal cords. An alternative technique is carefully to pass the laryngoscope into the proximal oesophagus and then draw back gradually to reveal the larynx.

Infants over 6 months and older children. In children over 6 months of age, a pillow may be required to provide some flexion of the neck. A laryngoscope with an adult blade (Macintosh) is frequently used, with the tip inserted anterior to the epiglottis at the base of the tongue. The laryngoscope should be lifted (not levered) to visualize the larynx. Although infant Macintosh blades are available, these have a wide cross-section and may impair the view of the larynx.

The tracheal tube should be inserted under direct vision between the vocal cords, and the laryngoscope carefully withdrawn while continuing to hold on to the tracheal tube at the mouth end. In children where a cuffed tube has been used (>8 years), the cuff should be inflated to provide an airtight seal.

Successful intubation. In all cases a catheter mount should be attached and ventilation commenced. Appropriate checks should then be made to ensure correct placement of the tube and ventilation of both lungs. Look for equal bilateral chest movement and listen for breath sounds bilaterally in the mid-axillary lines. Finally, listen over the epigastrium for gurgling sounds which may indicate oesophageal intubation. As in adults the ultimate check is to measure carbon dioxide in the expired gas.

Failed intubation. It is important not to persist with the attempt at intubation, and if it is not successful in the time that the rescuer can hold their breath (30 s), then the attempt should be abandoned. The child should be ventilated with 100% oxygen before further attempts are made. The complications and risks of intubation have already been detailed in Chapter 6.

9.5.3 Ventilation

Advanced ventilation consists of using either a self-inflating bag or a mechanical ventilator to deliver a high inspired oxygen concentration to the patient. An FIO_2 of 100% is the ideal.

Self-inflating bags are the most common devices used to ventilate apnoeic patients. Smaller volume bags of 240 ml and 500 ml are used for infants and children, respectively. They are fitted with a one-way valve to prevent rebreathing; this is pressure limited (45 cm H_2O) to prevent the lungs suffering from barotrauma due to over-enthusiastic ventilation.

These bags can be connected either to a face-mask of the appropriate size, or to the tracheal tube via a catheter mount. When used on their own the patient is ventilated with air (21% oxygen), but the FIO_2 can be raised to 50% by connecting an oxygen supply to an inlet adjacent to the air intake, and to 95% by using the addition of a reservoir bag.

It is important to remember that if a child-sized bag is not immediately available, an adult bag can be used if suitable adjustment is made in the tidal volume of gas delivered. The rates at which children should be ventilated are shown in Table 9.2.

Table 9.2   Ventilation rates

Age	Ventilatory rate/min
Neonates (less than 1 month)	60
Infant (less than 1 year)	30–40
1–8 years	20–30
>8 years	16
Adult	12

Mechanical ventilators can also be used to ventilate children of all ages. However, they are very powerful and if set incorrectly can deliver very large volumes of gas. Over-ventilation can impair cardiac function and may cause severe pulmonary barotrauma. On the whole these devices are best left to the experts who are familiar with them. Other problems associated with ventilation are discussed in Chapter 6.

Whichever method of advanced ventilation is used, it is important to check that the lungs are being adequately ventilated by looking for chest movement and listening for breath sounds.

9.5.4 The surgical airway

9.5.4.1 Needle cricothyroidotomy

Cricothyroidotomy is a 'technique of failure', and as such should only be used when all other means of obtaining an airway have failed. This situation usually occurs following laryngeal obstruction from a foreign body, inflammation or tumour, or following major trauma. Although cricothyroidotomy is rarely needed, it can be life-saving, and must be performed promptly when indicated. The technique is simple in concept but far from easy in practice, and not without hazard.

When possible, place the child in a supine position and extend the neck. If time allows the neck should be prepared with antiseptic. The cricothyroid membrane should be identified by palpation of the recess between the thyroid and cricoid cartilages, it should be stabilized with the thumb and index finger of the left hand. A cricothyroidotomy cannula or 14–16 g intravenous cannula, attached to a 5 ml syringe should be passed caudally through the membrane at a 45° angle; the syringe should be continually aspirated as the needle is advanced – air entering the syringe indicates that the needle is in the correct position. The cannula should then be slid off the needle further into the trachea. A further check should be made to ensure that air can still be aspirated. Ventilation can now be achieved by connecting an oxygen supply to the hub of the cannula, via a Y-connector as for an adult. It is not possible to ventilate adequately using a self-inflating bag through such a small cannula, since the pressures required for inflation are too high.

This technique is a temporizing measure for, although oxygenation can be achieved, carbon dioxide will accumulate, rendering the child acidotic. Urgent arrangements must be made to perform a definitive tracheostomy.

Needle cricothyroidotomy is to be preferred to surgical cricothyroidotomy in children under 12 years old, since damage to the cricoid cartilage (which is the only complete ring of cartilage supporting the trachea) is usually avoided.

9.6 THE MANAGEMENT OF CARDIAC ARREST

Cardiac arrest has occurred when there are no palpable central pulses. Basic life support with optimal oxygenation (preferably by intubation and ventilation) and with chest compressions must be established immediately. Chest compressions must not be interrupted for more than 10 s until satisfactory cardiac output has been restored, except to defibrillate.

The following arrest rhythms are discussed in this section:

Asystole
Ventricular fibrillation
Electromechanical dissociation

9.6.1 Asystole

This is the commonest arrest rhythm in children since the response of the young heart to prolonged, severe hypoxia and acidosis is progressive bradycardia leading to asystole (Figure 9.11).

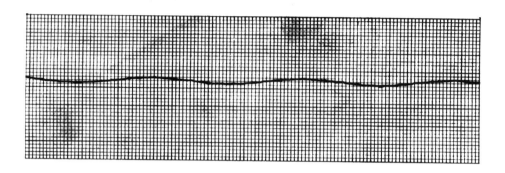

**Fig. 9.11
Asystole**

The algorithm for management of asystole in a child is shown in Figure 9.12.

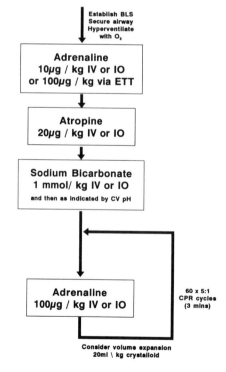

**Fig. 9.12
Algorithm for
management of
asystole in
children**

Adrenaline is the-first line drug. It is given initially in a dose of 10 µg/kg (0.1 ml of 1:10 000 solution). It is best given through a central line, but if one is not in place it may be given through a peripheral or intra-osseous line followed by a normal saline flush (2–5 ml). If there is no circulatory access, adrenaline can be given via the ET tube at ten times the intravenous dose. The drug should be injected quickly down a narrow bore suction catheter beyond the tracheal end of the ET tube and then flushed in with 1 or 2 ml of normal saline. Ventilation should then continue. In patients with pulmonary disease or prolonged asystole, pulmonary oedema and intrapulmonary shunting may make the endotracheal route for drugs less effective. If there has been no clinical effect, further doses should be given intravenously once venous access has been secured, as adrenaline is the only drug that has been shown to be effective in asystole.

After 1 min, atropine should be given intravenously (20 µg/kg) or intratracheally (0.04 mg/kg).

Children with asystole are usually profoundly acidotic as their cardiac arrest has usually been preceded by respiratory arrest or shock. The efficacy of adrenaline is reduced in acidosis and therefore sodium bicarbonate should precede further doses of adrenaline. The dose for children is 1 mmol/kg (1 ml per kg of 8.4% solution). In neonates the 8.4% solution should be diluted to 4.2%. It should be administered in boluses, not run in through a burette. It must not be given in the same intravenous line as calcium because precipitation will occur. Sodium bicarbonate inactivates adrenaline and dopamine and therefore the line must be flushed with saline if these drugs are subsequently given. Bicarbonate may not be given by the intratracheal route. Arterial blood gases should be taken to monitor the effect.

If the first dose of adrenaline was unsuccessful, further doses are given every 60 CPR cycles. Evidence suggests that the outcome is very poor if there is no response to the second dose of adrenaline.

9.6.2 Ventricular fibrillation (Figure 9.13)

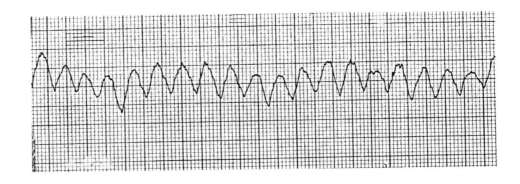

Fig. 9.13
Ventricular
fibrillation

This rhythm is uncommon in children but should be sought in those who are recovering from hypothermia, those poisoned by tricyclic antidepressants and those with cardiac disease. The algorithm for management of ventricular fibrillation (VF) in a child is shown in Figure 9.14.

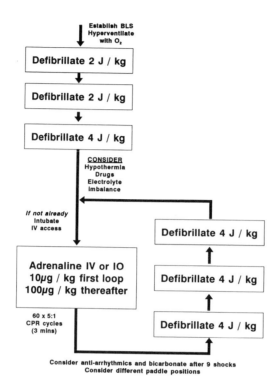

Fig. 9.14 Algorithm for management of VF in children

Electrical defibrillation should be carried out immediately. There is no place for a precordial thump in children. Paediatric paddles (4.5 cm diameter or equivalent area) should be used for children under 10 kg. One electrode is placed just below the right clavicle and the other in the left mid-clavicular line at the level of the xiphoid. If only adult paddles are available for an infant under 10 kg, one may be placed on the infant's back and one over the left lower part of the chest at the front.

The first two shocks should be at 2 J/kg, and the third at 4 J/kg. If these three shocks fail to produce defibrillation the patient should be hyperventilated (to increase pH), given adrenaline 10 µg/kg intravenously, and the shock (4 J/kg) repeated three times. This cycle is repeated with an adrenaline dose of 100 µg/kg. Different paddle positions or another defibrillator may be tried. Finally after nine shocks the anti-arrhythmic agents lignocaine, amiodarone or bretylium tosylate (5 mg/kg) may be used with further defibrillation attempts.

9.6.3 Electromechanical dissociation (EMD)

This is defined as absence of a palpable pulse, with recognizable complexes seen on the ECG monitor. The commonest cause in children is profound shock which makes the pulse difficult to feel. The algorithm for treatment of EMD in children is shown in Figure 9.15.

Fig. 9.15
Algorithm for
management of
EMD in children

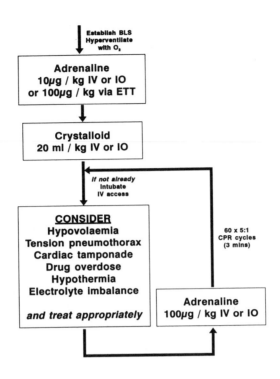

Adrenaline (10 µg/kg IV) should be given immediately. Rapid volume expansion with 20 ml/kg of crystalloid should then be commenced.

In patients who have suffered trauma, both cardiac tamponade and tension pneumothorax should be considered as causes of EMD, and should be treated as discussed in Chapter 8.

Very occasionally, intravenous calcium may be required in a patient with EMD due to hypocalcaemia, hyperkalaemia, hyper-magnesaemia or calcium channel blocker overdose. In this event patients should be treated with intravenous calcium chloride 10 mg/kg (0.1 ml/kg). The drug should be given slowly into a peripheral vein. Calcium may have serious toxic effects causing bradycardia, coronary artery spasm and myocardial irritability. It can cause severe local tissue damage if not given intravenously.

Adrenaline 100 µg/kg IV should be repeated every 60 CPR cycles.

9.7 OTHER DYSRHYTHMIAS IN CHILDHOOD

9.7.1 Supraventricular tachycardia (SVT)

This gives rise to a heart rate over 200 beats/min, and often up to 300 beats/min. The rhythm is regular and the QRS complexes are uniform in appearance. Each QRS is preceded by a P wave but this may not be apparent due to the tachycardia. This is shown in Figure 9.16.

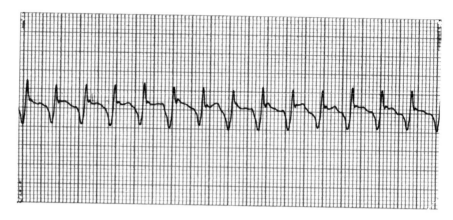

Fig. 9.16 Supraventricular tachycardia

The onset and cessation are sudden. The rhythm may last for minutes or up to several days. It is tolerated remarkably well by some children, but an infant may present with sweating, poor colour, peripheral vasoconstriction, hepatomegaly and other signs of cardiac failure. The SVT may rapidly degenerate into VF.

9.7.1.1 Unstable SVT

If the child is in shock use synchronized DC cardioversion. The first shock should be given at 0.5–1.0 J/kg, and further shocks should be given at 2.0 J/kg.

9.7.2 Ventricular tachycardia

This is defined as three or more ectopic ventricular beats, and is sustained if it continues for longer than 30 s. The rate varies between 120 and 250 beats/min (Figure 9.17).

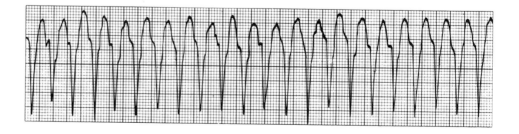

Fig. 9.17 Ventricular tachycardia

It is not a common presenting rhythm in children without an underlying congenital heart disorder, myocarditis or cardiomyopathy. It may occur after cardiac surgery. The onset may be sudden with rapid deterioration in tissue perfusion. This rhythm may degenerate into VF.

9.7.2.1 Unstable ventricular tachycardia

The unstable child should be given an unsynchronized DC shock. The first shock should be at 0.5–1.0 J/kg and should be followed by a bolus of IV lignocaine. Further shocks may be required, and should be given at 2.0 J/kg. An infusion of lignocaine may also be required.

9.7.3 Bradycardia in an unstable child

Treat hypoxia and shock. Give atropine 0.02 mg/kg (minimum 0.1 mg), then consider using adrenaline (0.01 mg/kg) and pacing.

9.8 POST-RESUSCITATION CARE

Once ventilation and spontaneous cardiac output have been established, it is essential that frequent clinical reassessment is carried out. Ventilatory and circulatory adequacy, and conscious level must be monitored to detect deterioration or improvement with therapy. All patients should be monitored as shown in Table 9.3.

Table 9.3 Methods of monitoring patients

Pulse rate and rhythm	ECG monitor
Oxygen saturation	Pulse oximeter
Core temperature	Low-reading thermometer
Blood pressure	Non-invasive monitor
Urine output	Urinary catheter
Arterial pH and gases	Arterial blood sample

Additionally, some patients will require CO_2 monitoring, invasive BP monitoring, and central venous pressure monitoring.

9.8.1 Airway and breathing

Most recently resuscitated children will have an impaired conscious level and depressed gag reflex. They should remain intubated and ventilated with a sufficient FIO_2 to maintain oxygen saturation above 95% and blood gases as normal as possible. Most survivors will be transferred to an ICU where ventilation can be adjusted as appropriate.

9.8.2 Circulation

Following cardiac arrest, cardiac output will usually be impaired by one or more of the following causes:

Underlying cardiac abnormality
Hypoxia, acidosis and toxins
Acid–base or electrolyte disturbance
Hypovolaemia

Arterial pH, oxygenation and electrolyte abnormalities should be identified and corrected. Hypoglycaemia should be sought and treated. Hypovolaemia should be treated by infusing 20 ml/kg of crystalloid or colloid. Following this, there may be a need for further circulatory expansion, inotropic drug support of the myocardium or vasodilatation of the circulatory system.

The placement of a central venous pressure (CVP) line will assist in deciding whether to give more fluid, or inotropic support. The CVP can be used to assess the response to a fluid challenge. The CVP of a hypovolaemic patient will alter little with a fluid bolus, but in one who is normovolaemic, hypervolaemic or has cardiac failure, it will show a sustained rise. This may indicate the need for inotropic support of the patient with poor cardiac output.

The choice of inotrope will vary with the patients' needs. Adrenaline may be the best inotropic drug for the child with post-arrest myocardial depression. It is infused at a rate of 0.05 µg/kg/min to 0.1 µg/kg/min. Dopamine is useful in low doses (1–3 µg/kg/min) to improve renal perfusion but may not be effective as an inotropic agent (dose 5–10 µg/kg/min) in the exhausted myocardium. Dobutamine may help the patient with poor perfusion and normal blood pressure (dose 2.5–20 µg/kg/min)

9.8.3 Cerebral management

Hypoxia and ischaemia occurring before cardiac arrest may have already caused brain damage. It is important to avoid further damage during the post-resuscitation period. This can be achieved by the following measures:

Good oxygenation
Normal blood pressure and perfusion
Normal acid–base balance and electrolytes
Normal blood sugar
Normothermia
Avoid unpleasant procedures without analgesia
Reduce intracranial pressure:
    Elevate bed head to 30°
    Restrict fluids to 60% when well perfused

Hyperventilate to $PaCO_2$ 28 mmHg (3.7 kPa)
Mannitol 500 mg/kg IV (if deteriorating neurologically)

9.8.4 Other considerations

Hypothermia. Sick or injured children become cold easily. Keep the child covered or under an infrared heater and monitor rectal temperature.

Hypoglycaemia. Sick infants have poor glycogen stores: glucose may need to be given during the course of CPR as indicated by stick tests. The dose is 0.5 g/kg IV.

9.8.5 When to stop resuscitation

If there has been no detectable signs of cardiac output and no evidence of cerebral activity despite 30 min CPR, it is reasonable to stop resuscitation. The decision will be taken by the team leader.

The exception is the hypothermic patient in whom resuscitation must continue until the patient has a core temperature of at least 32°C.

FURTHER READING

Morton, R. and Phillips, B. (1992) *Accidents and Emergencies in Children*. Oxford University Press, Oxford

Advanced Life Support Group (1992) *APLS (UK) Student Manual*.

Annex A
Equipment and technique for tracheal intubation of children

EQUIPMENT

1. Laryngoscope: choice of straight blade (e.g. Miller, Seward) or curved blade (Macintosh)
2. Tracheal tubes: for children over 1 year size calculated from:
   internal diameter (mm) = age in years/4 + 4
   length (cm) = age in years/2 + 12
   1 month to 1 year, 3–3.5 mm diameter, 12 cm in length
   one tube 0.5 mm smaller than calculated
   one tube 0.5 mm larger than calculated
   uncuffed tubes in children less than 8 years.
3. Catheter mount, to attach to ventilating device
4. Lubricant
5. Magills forceps
6. Introducer
7. Adhesive tape for securing tube
8. Ventilator
9. Suction

TECHNIQUE

1. Check equipment function, particularly: laryngoscope, suction, ventilation device
2. Choose correct size tracheal tube: length, diameter, cuff integrity
3. Preoxygenate the patient
4. Correct positioning of head
5. Laryngoscopy: holding laryngoscope correctly, correct use
6. Intubation: accomplished in <30 s from 'mask off'. If intubation attempt fails, re-establish ventilation with bag–valve–mask
7. Correct attachment of ventilating device
8. Ability to check correct positioning of tracheal tube and sequence of events if negative.

Annex B
Intra-osseous infusion

Intra-osseous infusion can be achieved effectively in less time and with less skill than is required to carry out a venous cut-down.

MINIMUM EQUIPMENT

Alcohol swabs
18 g needle at least 1.5 cm in length
5 ml syringe
50 ml syringe
Infusion fluid

PROCEDURE

1. Identify the infusion site. Fractured bones should be avoided, as should limbs with fractures proximal to the possible sites. The landmarks are: (i) tibial – anterior surface, 2–3 cm below the tibial tuberosity; and (ii) femoral – anterior surface, 3 cm above the lateral condyle. The tibial approach is shown in Figure 9.18.

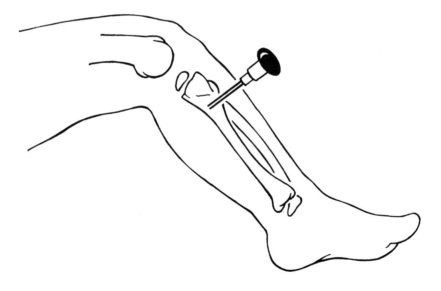

Fig. 9.18 Tibial technique for intra-osseous infusion

2. Clean the skin over the chosen site.
3. Insert the needle at 90° to the skin.
4. Apply pressure until a give is felt as the needle penetrates the cortex.
5. Attach the 5 ml syringe and aspirate to confirm correct positioning.
6. Attach the filled 50 ml syringe and push in the infusion fluid in boluses.

Practical skill station
Intra-osseous access

AIMS

To reinforce practically the knowledge of intra-osseous access gained in theoretical sessions.

To allow candidates to practice the procedure involved in intra-osseous access.

TEACHING TECHNIQUE

The technique is described and demonstrated using chicken thighs and an intra-osseous needle. Candidates are then allowed to practice.

TESTING

Candidates are informally assessed during this skill station. There is no formal assessment.

— 10 —
Special situations

Objectives

After studying this chapter you should be able to:

- Understand the variations in basic life support necessary in some special situations

- Understand the variations in advanced cardiac life support necessary in some special situations

- Understand the variations in post-resuscitation care necessary in some special situations

- Given a simulated patient model, demonstrate the correct application of these variations during resuscitation

---

Each patient with cardiac dysfunction or cardiorespiratory arrest is different, but the vast majority can be treated successfully by proper application of the appropriate protocols. However certain special situations require that modifications are made to some aspects of care. This part of the manual deals with some of these situations. These are:

Near drowning
Hypothermia
Pregnancy
Drug overdoses
Trauma
Electrical injury
Smoke inhalation

Each is covered in the same way. First, some background information is given. Second, under the heading 'Special considerations', the reasons for the particular problems of the situation are stated. In this section and in the following two sections ('Basic life support' and 'Advanced life support') these problems are dealt with in the familiar 'ABC' manner. Finally any changes necessary in the post-resuscitation care phase are noted.

If a heading does not appear then management is as per standard protocols.

10.1 NEAR DROWNING

10.1.1 Incidence

Near drowning is defined as an episode of suffocation by submersion followed by at least transient recovery. Its true UK incidence is unknown. However, there are 700 drowning episodes per year and, if the proportion of drowning to near drowning is the same as that in the USA, this suggests some 7700 cases. All ages are affected but it is most common in the second decade and in children under 4.

10.1.1.1 Aetiology and mechanism

Drowning in deep water may result from inability to swim or from exhaustion compounded by hypothermia. Trauma, especially to the cervical spine may render even the strongest swimmers liable to drowning, as may air emboli in scuba divers. Medical conditions such as epilepsy, hypoglycaemia, and intoxication with drugs or alcohol can cause drowning even in shallow water. Non-accidental submersion may occur, especially in children.

During a drowning episode water enters the airway and breathing stops, but the heart continues to beat and maintain cerebral perfusion for some time. Eventually the circulatory system fails and the patient has a cardiac arrest. The continued cardiac output following the cessation of breathing, coupled with rapid hypothermia may explain why some patients (especially children) can survive neurologically intact after long periods of submersion.

The main causes of late death in near drowning episodes are respiratory failure and ischaemic brain damage.

10.1.2 Special considerations

The clinical picture seen in near drowning is not affected by whether submersion was in salt or fresh water.

Safety. The water is dangerous both for the victim and for the rescuer.

A. There is a high incidence of neck injuries associated with drowning.

B. Draining water from the lungs makes little difference to the oxygen uptake but it does delay treatment and potentially jeopardizes an unstable neck.

Water enters some of the alveoli and washes out surfactant. Atelectasis results, along with ventilation-perfusion mismatch and damage to the alveolar-capillary membrane. Pulmonary oedema occurs in 75% of cases as a consequence of the surfactant loss, direct pulmonary injury, inflammatory contaminants in the water and cerebral hypoxia.

C. Hypothermia can occur, with consequent inability to feel central pulses even if they are present.

General. A combined respiratory and metabolic acidosis is common immediately after near drowning. However, by the time the patient reaches the emergency department, spontaneous respiration may already have been started. If breathing is adequate at this stage only the metabolic acidosis will remain.

The electrolyte disturbance, following the water absorption, is usually minor and rarely clinically significant.

Occasionally fresh water absorption can lead to anaemia due to haemolysis.

Renal failure can appear as a late consequence of hypoxia, hypotension, lactic acidosis and myoglobinuria.

Death cannot be declared until basic and advanced life support have been continued, without success, for 45 min and the core temperature is over 32°C. A longer time should be allowed for children.

10.1.3 Basic life support

Although life support can be rendered in water it is much more efficient (and safer for the rescuer) when administered on land.

SAFE. No untoward risks should be taken during the rescue, and all available aids (such as flotation devices) should be used.

Care must be taken to prevent exacerbation of any cervical injury by maintaining in-line stabilization of the neck. This should be continued even when the patient is being turned to clear away any vomitus.

B. Mouth to nose or mouth to mouth resuscitation can be started immediately, but all effort should be made to get the patient quickly from the water. Time should not be wasted attempting to drain water from the lungs.

10.1.4 Advanced life support

A. In-line cervical stabilization is maintained while the airway is reassessed and secured, and during intubation if this is required.

C. Usually volume support is not critical in these patients so that any infusion should initially be slow.

General. A low reading thermometer should be used to assess core temperature, and therapy for hypothermia commenced as discussed in the appropriate section.

10.1.5 Post-resuscitation care

A full examination is required to rule out associated injuries, including a pneumothorax and air emboli in divers.

A nasogastric tube and urinary catheter should be inserted if the patient is not fully conscious.

A chest radiograph is needed in all cases of near drowning because it does have a predictive value. Almost 50% of patients with an abnormal chest X-ray will require intubation and ventilation. The film may show perihilar infiltrates or pulmonary oedema.

Fever is common in the first few hours, but systemic infection should be suspected if a pyrexia develops after 24 h. Once blood cultures have been taken, intravenous antibiotics can then be started with the chosen agent being effective against Gram negative organisms. Prophylactic antibiotics and steroids are not required but regular tracheal cultures and blood for cultures, electrolytes and white cell counts should be taken.

Patients who have nearly drowned can be divided into three groups. These groups and their appropriate treatment are shown below:

1. Fully conscious, no respiratory distress, insignificant history of immersion. Discharged home after 6 h if there are no abnormalities found on examination of the chest, and there is a normal chest X-ray and arterial blood gases (ABG) result when the patient is breathing room air.
2. Conscious, mild/moderate respiratory distress. Require overnight observation in hospital. Provided there is no spinal injury, these patients should be managed on their side because they have a significant chance of vomiting.
3. Apnoeic, with a palpable pulse. Require admission to the intensive care unit with intubation, mechanical ventilation, haemodynamic monitoring and plasma expansion.

10.2 HYPOTHERMIA

Hypothermia has occurred when the core temperature falls below 35°C. It may complicate cardiac dysfunction arising from other causes, or may itself give rise to dysfunction. Hypothermia is divided into three grades according to the core temperature, as shown in Table 10.1.

Table 10.1 Grades of hypothermia, according to core temperature

Grade	Temperature (°C)
Mild	32–35
Moderate	30–32
Severe	<30

10.2.1 Aetiology and mechanism

Hypothermia can arise because of increased heat loss, decreased heat production, severe underlying disease, or from a combination of these mechanisms. Common causes underlying these are shown in Table 10.2.

Table 10.2 Causes of hypothermia

Increased heat loss	Decreased heat production	Underlying disease
Conduction:	Unconsciousness	Pancreatitis
Cold immersion	Hypothyroidism	
	Hypopituitarism	Bowel perforation
	Hypoglycaemia	
Convection:	Hypoadrenalism	Pneumonia
High winds	Old age	
Skin diseases	Children	
Burns	Hypothalamic lesion	
Vasodilatation:		Acute renal failure
Alcohol		
Drugs		
Infection		
Skin diseases		

The body has several protective mechanisms to prevent hypothermia developing should the environmental temperature fall. These involve reducing heat loss from the skin surface by vasoconstriction and behavioural responses (such as putting on more clothes). Heat production can also be enhanced by increasing metabolic rate and shivering.

If the environmental conditions overwhelm the normal protective mechanisms or these mechanisms fail, the core temperature will fall. The victim will then demonstrate signs and symptoms which are a combination of both the low temperature itself and the homeostatic mechanisms, as summarized in Table 10.3.

Table 10.3 Signs of hypothermia by severity

Mild	Moderate	Severe
Pale cold skin	Pale cold skin	Pale cold skin
Shivering	No shivering	No shivering
Tachycardia	Bradycardia	Bradycardia
Hypertension	Hypotension	Hypotension
Tachypnoea	Bradypnoea	Hypoventilation
	Confused/combative	Stupor/coma
		Areflexic
		Oliguria
		Arrhythmias
		AF
		Nodal/block
		VEs
		VF
		Asystole

10.2.2 Special considerations

A. With a fall in the consciousness level the cough and gag reflexes become impaired, thus aspiration pneumonia is more common.

B. As the core temperature falls there is a leftward shift in the oxyhaemoglobin dissociation curve, making oxygen release to tissues more difficult.

C. A 'cold diuresis' with subsequent hypovolaemia can occur because of an impairment of renal concentrating ability. This is aggravated by a plasma shift into the extravascular space.

Caution is needed with regard to the rate of fluid administration because the cold myocardium does not tolerate excessive fluid loads.

With a progressive fall in core temperature sinus bradycardia gives way to atrial fibrillation with a slow ventricular response. Eventually ventricular fibrillation and ultimately asystole occur. Furthermore, in severe hypothermia the myocardium can become very sensitive to the mildest of stimuli, such as simply moving the patient. Thus inappropriate cardiac massage can precipitate ventricular fibrillation which is resistant to electrical therapy until the core temperature is elevated.

General. The immobile, hypothermic patient is liable to develop rhabdomyolysis with acute tubular necrosis. Thrombosis can occur with subsequent embolic complications.

10.2.3 Treatment of hypothermia

Mild hypothermia can be treated by passive external rewarming alone. Moderate hypothermia is treated by this technique, together with the cautious infusion of warm saline. Severe hypothermia is treated by active external rewarming; active internal rewarming may be necessary in some cases. These methods are discussed below.

10.2.3.1 Passive rewarming

This method enables patients to rewarm themselves using their own metabolism. The patient is protected from the hostile environment, wet clothes are removed, and the skin is dried. Warm blankets are then used for insulation. The aim is to elevate the temperature by 0.5°C per hour.

10.2.3.2 Warm saline infusion

An intravenous infusion is started and warm saline administered to prevent any further heat loss. Caution is needed with regard to the rate of fluid administered.

10.2.3.3 Active external rewarming

This method is *inappropriate* until the core temperature is above 30°C. It is usually achieved by placing the patient in a warm bath. Close monitoring is essential since the peripheral vasodilatation that results increases the amount of cold blood returning to the core. The incidence of dysrhythmias may increase because of this. Furthermore vasodilatation can also lead to hypotension as well as acidosis from the wash-out of peripheral tissue lactic acid.

10.2.3.4 Active internal rewarming

This entails irrigation of the patient's core with warm fluid by gastric lavage, peritoneal lavage, a thoracic heat cradle or, in extreme situations, blood warming by haemodialysis or cardiopulmonary bypass. These techniques require varying degrees of expertise and equipment and all are better carried out in the intensive care unit. The more heroic measures should be reserved for persistent ventricular fibrillation or asystole.

10.2.4 Basic life support

Measures should be taken to prevent any further heat loss if possible. The patient should be handled as gently as possible throughout, to prevent the stimulation of ventricular fibrillation in the sensitive myocardium.

C. The pulse should be felt for 60 s. Only if no pulse is detected should external cardiac massage be started.

10.2.5 Advanced life support

Patients who have a palpable output but are severely hypothermic should be handled as gently as possible, in order to reduce the incidence of spontaneous dysrhythmia development.

C. Dysrhythmias, other than ventricular fibrillation, tend to correct themselves as the core temperature rises and require no specific treatment. Ventricular fibrillation may be resistant to cardioversion if the core temperature is less than 30°C. In this event a rapid rise in the core temperature is required (1–2°C per hour) and active internal rewarming techniques are appropriate.

General. The patient is not dead until both warm and dead. Advanced life support must be continued until the core temperature is at least 32°C. Only then can a definite diagnosis of death be made.

10.2.6 Post-resuscitation care

A chest X-ray and a 12-lead ECG are both essential. The latter may show 'J' waves (best seen in the V leads). These can occur at any subnormal temperature and so have no prognostic power.

The plasma electrolytes, alcohol, thyroid function, blood cultures, drug screen, glucose and ABG should be measured. The ABG analysis will need to be corrected for the low core temperature.

10.3 PREGNANCY

10.3.1 Incidence

Cardiac arrest occurs about once every 30 000 pregnancies.

10.3.2 Aetiology and mechanism

In addition to the usual causes, amniotic fluid embolus, eclampsia, and utero-placental haemorrhage may all result in cardiorespiratory arrest. Pulmonary embolus is more common.

10.3.3 Special considerations

In late pregnancy there are a number of anatomical and physiological changes which must be taken into account during attempted resuscitation.

A. The airway may be difficult to control due to neck obesity, breast enlargement and possible supra-glottic oedema. There is an increased risk of regurgitation and subsequent aspiration, both because of pressure on the stomach from the gravid uterus, and because of delayed gastric emptying.

B. Oxygen consumption is increased due to the metabolic demands of pregnancy, but chest compliance and functional residual capacity are decreased for mechanical reasons.

C. In the supine position the uterus compresses the inferior vena cava resulting in reduced venous return.

10.3.4 Basic life support

Since oxygen consumption is increased, the pregnant patient will develop cerebral hypoxia more rapidly than the non-pregnant. Basic life support should therefore be initiated as quickly as possible.

Cricoid pressure should be applied by an assistant while ventilating the patient. This will reduce the risk of aspiration of gastric contents.

C. Pressure on the inferior vena cave should be relieved to increase venous return, otherwise cardiac massage will not produce an adequate output. This can be achieved either by inclining the patient 30° laterally (using a wedge under the right side) (Figure 10.1), or by an assistant manually moving the uterus to the left and towards the head (Figure 10.2).

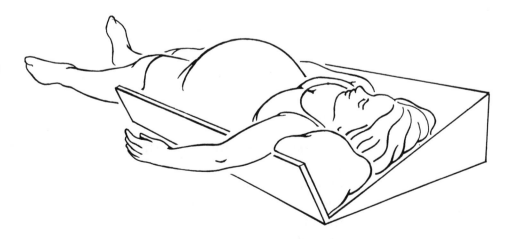

Fig. 10.1 The use of a resuscitation wedge

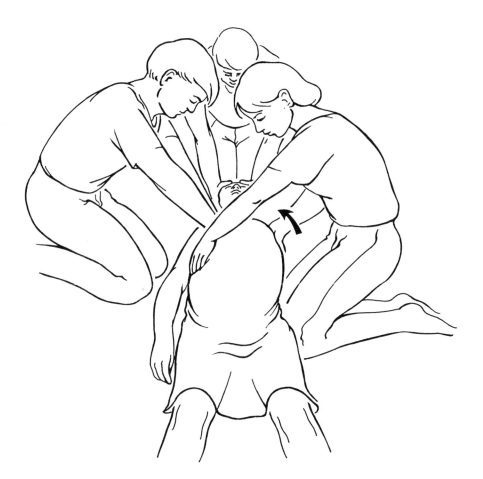

**Fig. 10.2
Manual uterine
displacement**

10.3.5 Advanced life support

Any obvious causes of the arrest, such as hypovolaemia or status epilepticus secondary to eclampsia, should be treated.

A. Cricoid pressure should be maintained until the airway is both controlled and protected.

Intubation is more difficult but should be attempted as soon as possible. It may prove impossible to insert a standard laryngoscope as the breasts can obstruct the handle. This problem can be overcome in one of two ways. Either a special laryngoscope is used, or the blade of a standard laryngoscope is put in the mouth and the handle attached afterwards.

C. Dysrhythmias should be treated according to standard protocols unless the patient has undergone epidural anaesthesia. In that situation the following modifications to drug protocols apply:

Adrenaline should be administered early to help counteract vasodilation.
Lignocaine should be avoided as cumulation with the anaesthetic agent used for the epidural may prove toxic. Bretylium tosylate is therefore the preferred drug for the treatment of refractory VF in this situation.

General. If resuscitation is unsuccessful after 5 min then emergency caesarian section should be performed. This improves the mother's chances of survival as the inferior vena cava is further decompressed, and also helps the foetus. ACLS should continue throughout surgery.

10.3.6 Post-resuscitation care

Surviving patients will all require urgent obstetric consultation, and paediatricians should be called to look after the child. Specific obstetric causes of the arrest should be sought and treated appropriately. Since aspiration of acid gastric contents is likely, the resulting chemical pneumonitis (Mendelsohn's syndrome) should be sought and treated.

10.4 DRUG OVERDOSES

10.4.1 Aetiology and mechanism

Cardiovascular collapse or cardiorespiratory arrest may be caused by either an accidental or a deliberate drug overdose. In the older patient prescribed drugs are usually responsible, whereas in the younger patient either prescribed or 'street' drugs are seen. Alcohol is often a complicating factor. The identity of the abused substance must be ascertained as soon as possible, and the effects noted. This may allow appropriate treatment to be commenced early enough to prevent cardiac arrest. If arrest does occur, the usual treatment protocols may be inadequate.

10.4.2 Special considerations

A. Patients with an altered consciousness level may have an absent gag reflex, and therefore an inadequately protected airway.

B. Hypoxia potentiates the deleterious effects of any drug overdose, which causes embarrassment of the cardiovascular system. Oxygen is therefore a key treatment.

General. Hypoglycaemia can occur after overdosage, especially if alcohol is also involved. Blood glucose must always be measured early and any abnormalities promptly treated.

Combined drug overdoses may be more difficult to treat, and larger than normal doses of pharmaceutical agents may be required to achieve a desired effect.

10.4.3 Advanced life support

A. The gag reflex should be sought and the airway adequately protected if it is absent.

C. Apparent ventricular fibrillation may in fact be Torsades de Pointes. The former is a state of abnormal depolarization where lignocaine may be helpful after defibrillation. Torsades is a state of abnormal repolarization in which lignocaine may be counterproductive. Lignocaine prolongs repolarization, thus potentiating the primary electrical abnormality.

General. If indicated the residual drug should be eliminated from the stomach by lavage, and from the gut by administering activated charcoal. Lavage may cause excess vagal activity due to oropharyngeal stimulation, especially in beta-blocker overdoses.

10.4.4 Specific drugs

Opiates. There is little hope of resuscitating an opiate overdose without the administration of large quantities of naloxone. An intravenous dose of 0.4–1.6 mg should be given initially; this should be repeated at regular intervals throughout the resuscitation period.

The short half-life of naloxone requires that a continuous infusion be commenced when resuscitation is successful. An initial rate of 0.4–0.8 mg/h (in 5% dextrose) is used, and this is titrated to clinical effect. Intramuscularly administered naloxone has a longer half-life, and may be of use in the non-co-operative addict. Naloxone will, of course, precipitate an acute withdrawal state in such addicts.

Beta-blockers. The most severe effects of beta-blocker overdose (pallor, hypotension, bradycardia and hypoglycaemia) are associated with the least cardioselective drugs such as propranolol. Patients may respond to the standard bradycardia protocol, but if they don't intravenous glucagon should be given. The dose in adults is 5–10 mg stat, followed by an infusion at 1–5 mg/h. In children the doses are 0.15 mg/kg, and 0.05–0.1 mg/kg/h, respectively.

Tricyclic antidepressants. This group of drugs is particularly dangerous. They induce a state of cardiac irritability which may result in the development of a variety of drug-resistant, and often life-threatening, dysrhythmias. These may develop or recur for up to 24–36 h after ingestion. A prolonged QT interval is associated with a higher incidence of dysrhythmias.

Whatever the rhythm on the ECG, the initial treatment is 1–2 mmol/kg of sodium bicarbonate intravenously (50 ml 8.4% solution as an initial bolus for an adult). Even in VF, sodium bicarbonate should be given early, i.e. after the first three DC shocks. Further aliquots of 50 ml should be given until either the blood pH is 7.55 or the dysrhythmia has reverted to sinus rhythm.

Tricyclics can also cause fits and hyperthermia, both of which should be treated in the usual way.

Cardiac glycosides. Acute poisoning with cardiac glycosides causes a raised serum potassium and conduction abnormalities (mostly varying degrees of A-V block). Chronic poisoning is often associated with a low or normal serum potassium and, unusually, serious dysrhythmias such as VT or VF may develop, apparently aggravated by the hypokalaemia.

Digoxin. Only about 20% of an oral dose is absorbed, and it is 6–12 h before this is fixed in the tissues. If life-threatening dysrhythmias do occur they should be treated according to the usual protocols. In addition, digoxin-specific (Fab) antibodies should be given. It takes some 30–60 min for these to begin to reverse the signs of digoxin intoxication, and the peak effect is seen at 3 h. Every 40 mg of antibodies binds 0.6 mg of digoxin; consequently the dose required varies with the size of the overdose.

Digoxin-specific (Fab) antibodies are kept in regional and sub-regional centres only, but are available urgently on demand. Any poisons unit will be able to give the name of the nearest hospital that can supply them, and any contact names and numbers that are required.

10.5 TRAUMA

10.5.1 Aetiology and mechanism

Trauma can cause cardiac dysrhythmia or arrest in a number of ways. Direct injury to the heart may be so severe as to cause disruption, which is invariably fatal, or may precipitate cardiac tamponade, or cause cardiac contusion with its attendant risks of dysrhythmias. Injuries to the chest may cause arrest secondary to hypoxia, or may cause restriction of the mediastinum as in tension pneumothorax. Finally, severe bleeding may cause hypovolaemic arrest.

All of the treatable causes of traumatic cardiac dysrhythmia and arrest are dealt with elsewhere in this text, and are not dealt with again here. Reference may be found to them as follows:

Hypoxia: Chapter 6
Tension pneumothorax: Chapter 8
Cardiac contusion: Chapter 7
Cardiac tamponade: Chapter 8
Hypovolaemia: Chapter 8

10.6 ELECTRICAL INJURIES

10.6.1 Aetiology and mechanism

Electrical injuries occur either because of contact with power sources, or because of lightning strike.

Power sources. Dry skin offers high resistance to electricity. However, skin that has been moistened with water, sweat, or other conductive fluid has a much reduced resistance. The injury caused depends on the nature and size of the current, the duration, the area exposed, and the path the current follows. DC is less dangerous than AC. AC currents of 25–300 Hz and 25–240 V tend to cause ventricular fibrillation if the path crosses the heart. If the voltage is over 1000 V respiratory paralysis is common. At intermediate currents, a mixed picture of dysrhythmia with respiratory insufficiency is likely.

Lightning. Lightning is a direct current which travels from thunderclouds to the ground at speeds of up to 1 million metres per second. It can attain voltages of more than 100 million volts and temperatures of up to 3000°C. Lightning injuries may be from direct strikes, splash from surrounding structures, or step voltage (the transmission of ground surface current through a circuit created by the victim's legs).

Cardiac arrest may occur as the result of sudden cardiac standstill caused by the huge DC countershock of the lightning strike. Both ventricular fibrillation and asystole have been reported. Respiratory arrest is the commonest cause of death following lightning strike, and may occur due to brain stem shock or contusion, or because of respiratory muscle paralysis. Respiratory arrest may be complicated by cardiac arrest either because of simultaneous cardiac standstill, or because of secondary hypoxic effects. Myocardial infarction may occur as an acute complication.

10.6.2 Special considerations

In the case of injury from power sources, diagnosis is usually from the history. If lightning strike has occurred and no history is available, characteristic 'flashover' burn injury patterns may aid diagnosis:

1. Linear: superficial and partial thickness, beginning at the head and neck, and flowing in a branching pattern down the chest and legs.
2. Feathering: these are the cutaneous imprints of electron showers. They appear like a delicately branching fern.
3. Punctate: full or partial thickness, circular, in clusters that form starburst patterns.

Safety. Electrical current can cause continued injury to the patient, and significant injury to the rescuer.

A. Electrical burns to the face and airway may occur.

10.6.3 Basic life support

SAFE. The victim should be freed from the current at once by turning off the power.

It is essential that the rescuer is protected while this is being done

10.6.4 Advanced life support

A. If facial burns have occurred intubation may be difficult. It is important to achieve definitive airway care early, as difficulty will increase with time. Specialist anaesthetic help should be sought in this situation, and surgical control of the airway may be necessary.

10.6.5 Post-resuscitation care

If resuscitation is successful (return of spontaneous circulation) the patient should be maintained on a ventilator for 12–24 h before weaning is attempted. This is to allow time for spontaneous respiratory activity to return. Cardiac monitoring should continue throughout this period. Fixed dilated pupils are of no prognostic significance following electrical injury.

10.7 SMOKE INHALATION

10.7.1 Aetiology and mechanism

Smoke inhalation may cause three types of injury:

1. Thermal injury to the airways
2. Chemical injury to the airways and lungs
3. Systemic poisoning

Agents involved in chemical injury include acrolein (a highly reactive aldehyde) from wood and petroleum products, hydrochloric acid from polyvinyl chloride, toluene di-isocyanate from polyurethane, and nitrogen dioxide from cars and agricultural wastes. Carbon monoxide formed during incomplete combustion, and cyanide found during house fires both cause systemic poisoning.

A combination of thermal injury and poisoning, together with lowering of inspired oxygen levels during the fire, can result in hypoxic cardiorespiratory arrest.

10.7.2 Special considerations

All patients presenting following a fire in an enclosed space should be suspected of suffering from smoke injury. Carbonaceous sputum and perioral burns also strongly suggest this diagnosis.

Safety. Continued exposure to smoke can cause injury to the patient and can harm the rescuer.

A. Airway management may be complicated by perioral burns and thermal burns to the airways themselves.

B. Carbon monoxide poisoning may occur. The high affinity of carboxyhaemoglobin for oxygen further exacerbates tissue hypoxia. Carboxyhaemoglobin levels will start to decrease once the victim is removed from the toxic environment, even if they are breathing air, and this should be borne in mind. Stat estimations should be interpreted as shown in Table 10.4.

Table 10.4 Stat estimations of carboxyhaemoglobin level

	Carboxyhaemoglobin level (%)
Non-smokers	<1
Smokers	4–6
Significant exposure	>10

At levels above 50%, myocardial infarction may occur, especially in individuals with pre-existing ischaemic disease. Alkalosis and hypothermia decrease the dissociation of carbon monoxide and should be avoided.

10.7.3 Basic life support

SAFE. The victim should be removed from the smoke-filled environment as soon as possible. It may be necessary for a rescuer wearing breathing apparatus to do this.

10.7.4 Advanced life support

A. If perioral, neck, or airway burns have occurred intubation may be difficult. It is important to achieve definitive airway care early, as difficulty will increase with time. Specialist anaesthetic help should be sought in this situation, and surgical control of the airway may be necessary.

B. Urgent estimation of carboxyhaemoglobin levels should be undertaken. Care should be taken not to cause respiratory alkalosis by hyperventilation.

General. Hypothermia should be corrected as discussed in the relevant section.

10.7.5 Post-resuscitation care

If spontaneous respiration returns and carbon monoxide levels are not raised, close monitoring for late-onset bronchospasm and pulmonary oedema should be undertaken. This may occur up to 24 h after exposure. If carbon monoxide levels are significantly raised, ventilation with 100% oxygen should be continued at least until levels are within the normal range. The use of hyperbaric oxygen, although theoretically desirable, may be impracticable in the ventilated patient because of the need for intense monitoring. However, local specialist advice should be sought as facilities that allow this may exist.

11

Post-resuscitation care

Objectives

After studying this chapter you should be able to:

- Understand the spectrum of expected outcomes

- Understand the spectrum of care needed

- Understand the approach to patient assessment

- Understand the initiation of diagnostic work-up

- Understand the basics of CCU and ICU treatment

- Understand the pointers to likely neurological outcome

11.1 SPECTRUM OF OUTCOMES

The return of a spontaneous circulation does not necessarily mean the end of a successful resuscitation: more likely, it marks the start of a long and difficult post-resuscitation care phase. The aim of resuscitation is to produce a fully conscious, neurologically intact patient who has a spontaneous and stable cardiac rhythm with adequate cardiorespiratory function.

Following early and effective resuscitation after primary cardiac arrest the patient may recover almost immediately. If stable, these patients can usually be transferred to a Coronary Care Unit (CCU) for observation.

More frequently, however, resuscitation is more prolonged and the patient will remain obtunded. Usually mechanical ventilation is needed due to fractured ribs or inadequate respirations and often drug therapy is needed to maintain a circulation. These patients require transfer to an Intensive Care Unit (ICU) when as stable as is possible, for invasive haemodynamic monitoring and ventilation.

11.2 INITIAL ASSESSMENT

11.2.1 History prior to transfer

A careful evaluation should be obtained prior to transfer, including any antecedent history. In hospital, if the patient is found to have an end-stage or terminal condition it may be deemed correct to leave the patient on the ward and to withhold further therapy.

A history of overdose, especially of tricyclic antidepressants or narcotics, is valuable.

The possibility of hypoglycaemic or hypoxic-induced arrest must be ascertained, and consideration given to whether the cardiac arrest was preceded by an obvious neurological event such as a stroke.

An estimate of the duration of arrest prior to starting resuscitation is sometimes available and is prognostically important. The duration of CPR and drugs given should be obtained.

11.2.2 Examination prior to transfer

Prior to transfer, rapid examination of the patient will rule out easily correctable problems and establish a baseline.

1. Examine the respiratory system. Rule out pneumothorax and ascertain position of the endotracheal tube by listening for breath sounds and watching chest movements. Commonly the endotracheal tube is inserted too far (more than 22 cm on average) and usually enters the right main bronchus so that air entry is reduced on the left. Often crepitus from fractured ribs will be apparent at this stage. Place a chest tube if necessary.

2. Examine the cardiovascular system. Listen for heart sounds and palpate the major pulses. Look for grossly distended or absent neck veins which may alert you to tamponade, acute right heart failure (pulmonary embolus) or hypovolaemia. Absence of femoral, but presence of brachial pulses should raise the possibility of an abdominal aortic aneurysm. Severe hypovolaemia following haemorrhage from trauma, ectopic pregnancy or ruptured aortic aneurysm requires rapid fluid infusion. Cardiac tamponade requires needle aspiration.

3. Look at the ECG monitor. Tall T waves may indicate hyperkalaemia seen in renal failure or crush injury. Treatment involves bolus doses of intravenous calcium (5 mmol) and administration of a dextrose/insulin infusion. Arrhythmias fol-

lowing tricyclic poisoning need expert attention but consider hyperventilation, bicarbonate, magnesium and pacing.

4. Carry out a limited neurological assessment. Note the Glasgow Coma Score, pupil size and corneal reflex. Look for obvious lateralizing signs by changes in limb tone or movement. Narcotic overdose responds to intravenous naloxone and benzodiazepine overdose to flumazenil.

5. Examine the abdomen. This may detect a distended stomach or other obvious swelling such as aortic aneurysm. Obvious gastric dilatation should be decompressed by passage of a nasogastric tube if possible.

11.3 CARE OF THE OPTIMALLY RESUSCITATED PATIENT

Oxygen should be given by face-mask. A flow of 4 l/min gives an inspired concentration of about 24%–30%. ECG monitoring should be instituted and intravenous access secured. Intravenous analgesia should be given (such as morphine 2 mg repeated as necessary), especially in myocardial infarction. Anti-arrhythmics such as lignocaine should be continued and the patient transferred to the CCU. There, further management of arrhythmias will be undertaken if needed and any further diagnostic work-up completed. The patient is closely observed for any deterioration in organ function.

11.4 CARE OF THE PATIENT REQUIRING ORGAN SUPPORT

Profound global ischaemia as occurs during cardiac arrest leads to rapid depletion of intracellular energy stores, and depolarization of cell membranes with potassium loss and calcium influx. There is loss of cellular and organ function which paradoxically may worsen in the early recovery phase, the so-called 'reperfusion' injury.

From a practical point of view, intermittent positive pressure ventilation should be continued with 100% oxygen and ECG monitoring commenced. Anti-arrhythmic and vasoactive therapies may be needed to stabilize the patient prior to and during transport to the ICU. Because the patient will be on mechanical ventilation, sedative and paralysing drugs may be needed. On ICU the diagnostic examination and investigations will be completed and treatments for organ support instituted.

11.5 DIAGNOSTIC WORK-UP

Immediate investigations include a 12-lead ECG, chest X-ray, arterial blood gases, electrolyte, creatinine and blood sugar estimations. A lactate measurement can give some estimate of the degree of tissue hypoxia. Central venous blood gases are taken if a central line has been inserted.

The chest X-ray is scrutinized for fractures. Broken ribs may often be visible on the straight chest X-ray but if a fractured sternum is suspected a lateral film may be necessary for confirmation. Pneumothoraces are obvious if very large, but on supine films can be difficult to see, even for the experienced clinician. Parenchymal lung injury or aspiration are not uncommon during resuscitation. A large heart or widened mediastinum should be noted but cardiac tamponade is not always obvious on chest X-ray. The position of the endotracheal tube, nasogastric tube and any intravascular lines or pacing wire should be confirmed.

The 12-lead ECG is often necessary to distinguish ventricular from supraventricular arrhythmias, although in the immediate post-myocardial infarction period most are ventricular in origin. Changes may also be seen as a result of hyperkalaemia (tall T waves), pulmonary embolus with a right ventricular strain pattern (S wave lead I, Q wave and T wave inversion in lead III, rSR and T wave inversion in V_1) or of myocardial infarction (ST elevation, Q waves).

11.6 HAEMODYNAMIC MONITORING

Non-invasive and clinical assessments of cardiac function are inaccurate in at least 30%–50% of patients admitted to Intensive and Coronary Care Units. Empirical therapy may be ineffectual or hazardous if a correct haemodynamic assessment has not been made.

11.6.1 Measurement of blood pressure

It is well known that, in patients with a high systemic vascular resistance, cuff blood pressure may be almost inaudible and peripheral pulses almost impalpable despite there being a normal central arterial pressure. Therefore a large artery such as the femoral or brachial is cannulated for blood pressure recording.

11.6.2 Measurement of cardiac filling pressures and cardiac output

A central venous pressure line is useful for infusing vasoactive drugs and reflects right ventricular function in relation to venous return. It cannot be used reliably to estimate left ventricular function.

Because of intense vasoconstriction, a normal blood pressure does not always mean there is an adequate cardiac output. It may therefore be necessary to use a pulmonary artery flotation catheter ('Swan-Ganz' catheter). This will allow measurement of pulmonary artery pressures, cardiac output and true mixed venous blood gases, and an estimate of left atrial pressure ('wedge pressure').

11.6.3 Measurement of oxygen transport variables

By combining measurements of the oxygen content in arterial and mixed venous blood with the cardiac output, it is possible to estimate the amount of oxygen transported to and consumed by the tissues. Shock is now defined as a failure to deliver an adequate supply of oxygen to the tissues and not simply in terms of a low blood pressure. Measurement and manipulation of oxygen transport variables is considered central to the rational treatment of patients in shock.

11.7 CARDIOVASCULAR SUPPORT

Following myocardial infarction the following values are associated with improved outcome: cardiac index (cardiac output/body surface area) >2.2 l/min/m^2 with wedge pressure <18 mmHg. Mean arterial pressure should preferably be near normal (80–100 mmHg) to maintain coronary artery perfusion pressure. In order to ensure adequate tissue oxygenation the mixed venous oxyhaemoglobin saturation (SvO_2) should be greater than 60%. On the ICU, fluids and vasoconstrictors are often needed to improve circulatory function, although vaso-dilators, diuretics and inotropes are frequently also given to patients following myocardial infarction.

11.8 RESPIRATORY SUPPORT

The airway must be secure and adequate ventilation is essential. In the majority of cases this will require endotracheal intubation and mechanical ventilation. The patient may need to be paralysed and sedated to avoid fighting the ventilator. Ventilate with 100% oxygen until arterial blood gases are measured and then adjust the inspired oxygen to keep the arterial PO_2 in the 12–15 kPa range. Continuous hyperventilation is not of major benefit and the $PaCO_2$ can be kept in the 4–5 kPa range. If hypoxia persists, positive end expiratory pressure (PEEP) may be necessary, but it is essential to measure cardiac filling pressures and cardiac output before therapeutic PEEP is added since, although the PaO_2 may improve, the cardiac output and hence oxygen delivery may fall.

11.9 RENAL SUPPORT

Following a period of hypotension and hypoxia renal function is likely to suffer. Following catheterization urine volumes are measured hourly, an output of at least 0.5 ml/kg/h and preferably 1 ml/kg/h is the goal. To some degree, this reflects adequate organ perfusion if mannitol or diuretics have not been given. Renal function is best optimized by ensuring adequate cardiorespiratory status as described above. The administration of diuretics to an oliguric patient who is hypovolaemic, hypotensive and hypoxic is illogical. Although frusemide and mannitol may have a place in ensuring adequate tubular flow, the use of these agents has not been shown to reverse acute renal dysfunction if hypotension and tissue hypoxia persist.

11.10 GASTROINTESTINAL SUPPORT

The gut as an organ also suffers from the effects of low cardiac output and from reperfusion injury. Treatment is as above and aims to maintain the delivery of well oxygenated blood to all parts of the gut. Gastric dilatation should be prevented by the use of a nasogastric tube, and stress ulcer prophylaxis should be considered. Early enteric feeding is beneficial to gut function.

11.11 NEUROLOGICAL SUPPORT

Cerebral perfusion pressure (CPP) is the difference between mean arterial pressure (MAP) and intracranial pressure (ICP):

$$CPP = MAP - ICP$$

It is important to maintain a normal or even high normal cerebral perfusion pressure. This is best achieved by minimizing known reasons for increased intracranial pressure such as hypercarbia, coughing or fighting the ventilator. The indiscriminate use of mannitol is not recommended unless intracranial pressure is being monitored. A normal or high normal mean arterial pressure should be maintained if this can be achieved without jeopardizing myocardial function. Increased cerebral metabolism should be avoided by treating any seizures that occur and reducing hyperpyrexia. Hyperglycaemia is harmful to brain tissue that is ischaemic and should be avoided.

11.11.1 Neurological outcome indicators

The brief neurological assessment carried out immediately post-resuscitation is of prognostic value although full neurological assessments are generally delayed until 6 and 24 h later to improve reproducibility.

Conscious level is assessed by the Glasgow Coma Score (GCS):

Eye opening

1. *Nil*
2. *To pain*
3. *To commands*
4. *Spontaneously*

Motor response

1. *Nil*
2. *Extends*
3. *Abnormal flexion*
4. *Withdraws*
5. *Localizes*
6. *Obeys commands*

Verbal

1. *Nil*
2. *Incomprehensible*
3. *Inappropriate*
4. *Confused*
5. *Orientated*

Patients in coma have a GCS of 7 or less. They fail to obey commands, express no sounds and do not open their eyes.

Hemisphere function is assessed by limb tone, power and reflexes to look for localizing signs.

Brain stem function is assessed by pupillary and corneal response, eye movements, cough and gag or grimace reflexes. The pupils are not useful immediately post-arrest as an indicator of cerebral dysfunction, because catecholamines and atropine are frequently given during CPR and can cause dilatation of the pupils.

It is important to rule out cerebral trauma, intoxication, severe sepsis or meningitis before making predictions of neurological outcome. The presence of seizures, which occur in approximately 25% of patients, is not of prognostic importance.

If CPR was initiated following a primary cardiac event then the coma is of a hypoxic/ischaemic nature. Only 10%–15% of patients remaining in coma for >6 h gain an independent existence and 20% will enter a persistent vegetative state.

By utilizing brain stem reflexes as well as the GCS one can be more certain of outcome. At 24 h, absent brain stem reflexes almost precludes a good recovery, but not, of course, survival!

12

Cardiopulmonary resuscitation: Putting it all together

Objectives

After studying this chapter you should be able to:

- Understand the sequence of management in cardiopulmonary resuscitation

- Understand the roles within the resuscitation team

- Understand the role and responsibilities of the team leader

- Given a simulated patient model, demonstrate the correct sequence of management

- Given a simulated patient model, demonstrate proficiency at team leadership

While the initial aim in the management of any life-threatening emergency is to preserve life, the true measure of success must surely be the discharge of a patient who is as well as, or better than, before. If a cardiac resuscitation attempt is to be successful to this degree, correct management must start immediately, and continue to be provided until the post-resuscitation care phase is finished. Failure to provide optimum care at any stage will lessen the chances of a favourable outcome. There are no second chances.

The earlier chapters in this manual have discussed both the background and therapeutic knowledge that are necessary to provide optimum care. The practical skills that are required have also been dealt with. Successful resuscitation, however, requires not only that those involved in the attempt possess both of these, but also that their knowledge and skills are applied quickly and appropriately. This chapter deals both with the correct application of knowledge and skills, and with the control of the resuscitation attempt.

12.1 THE SEQUENCE OF MANAGEMENT OF CARDIOPULMONARY RESUSCITATION

The ideal sequence for cardiac resuscitation is shown in Figure 12.1. This sequence is designed to optimize the outcome by ensuring both that diagnosis and basic life support precede advanced cardiac life support, and that advanced techniques and treatments are carried out in the most efficacious order. If more than one member of the resuscitation team is capable of performing advanced techniques, then some tasks may be carried out concurrently; however, the overall order should still be followed.

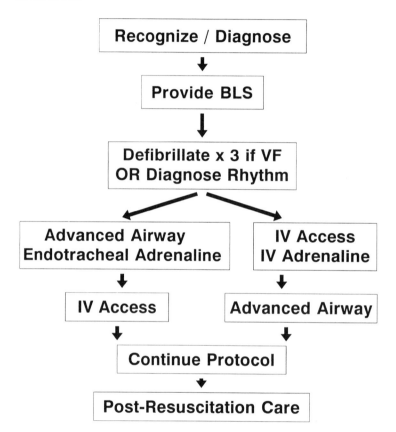

Fig. 12.1 The overall sequence of cardiac resuscitation

12.1.1 Recognition and diagnosis

It is essential that a cardiopulmonary collapse is recognized swiftly and diagnosed accurately, since these two steps must precede the administration of basic life support. Many people (even professional health care providers) have surprising difficulty in persuading themselves that a patient has suffered cardiopulmonary collapse; this is presumably because of the embarrassment they would feel if wrong. Since time to basic life support is so critical in determining outcome, every effort must be made to fight against this tendency 'to be absolutely sure'. By applying the methods of assessment discussed in Chapter 2 (the SAFE approach, evaluate ABC) these delays can be avoided. It is always better to overdiagnose and be embarrassed, than to underdiagnose and reduce the chances of a good outcome.

12.1.2 Basic life support

It is essential that basic life support is applied early and well, **and continued throughout the resuscitation attempt**. Cardiac and respiratory support should never be discontinued for more than 10 s (except during defibrillation) from the time the diagnosis is made, until either spontaneous circulation and breathing return, or the attempt at resuscitation is formally abandoned. Failure to provide continuous good basic life support greatly decreases the chance of a favourable outcome.

The techniques of basic life support are discussed in detail in Chapter 2.

12.1.3 Defibrillation and rhythm diagnosis

12.1.3.1 Defibrillation

Defibrillation is the single most efficacious treatment in adult cardiac arrest, since the majority of salvageable patients are suffering from ventricular fibrillation. Furthermore, as discussed in Chapter 1, the time to delivery of the first DC shock is critical in determining outcome. It follows, therefore, that defibrillation should be the first manoeuvre to be considered in the advanced cardiac life support of cardiac arrest.

In ventricular fibrillation and pulseless ventricular tachycardia three attempts at defibrillation should precede all other advanced interventions. If the rhythm appears to be asystole but ventricular fibrillation cannot be excluded, the same sequence should be followed. The pulse in the carotid artery should be checked for 5 s after each shock to assess whether spontaneous circulation has returned. Basic life support must be continued throughout without a break of more than 10 s, except during the delivery of the shock itself.

Since ventricular fibrillation is common and treatable, and time is important, 'blind defibrillation' (that is defibrillation carried out prior to monitoring of any sort) should be carried out in situations in which monitoring is unavailable. The use of paddle electrodes and the advent of automatic and semi-automatic defibrillators have made such circumstances very rare.

Defibrillation is discussed in detail in Annex A to Chapter 8.

12.1.3.2 Rhythm diagnosis

If ventricular fibrillation and pulseless ventricular tachycardia can be excluded, the rhythm should be diagnosed while airway control and/or vascular access are being achieved. It is important to make an accurate diagnosis of the rhythm as early as possible, so that the correct treatment protocol can be applied.

Dysrhythmia recognition is discussed in detail in Chapter 7.

12.1.4 Endotracheal intubation and vascular access

If immediate defibrillation is not indicated or has failed and adequate basic life support is being achieved using standard techniques, the next priority is to establish a route for drug administration. Since adrenaline is the first drug given in all the cardiac arrest protocols, and because this can be administered by either the intravenous or tracheal routes, either endotracheal intubation or central venous cannulation may be carried out at this stage. If the patient has not arrested, and does not therefore require intubation or a central venous line, peripheral intravenous access should be established.

The choice of initial route should be made by the team leader, taking into account both the condition of the patient and the skills of team members. In general, if skills are limited and procedures cannot be carried out concurrently, patients need the airway protection offered by a cuffed endotracheal tube before they require central venous access. Thus intubation is often carried out first, and the initial dose of adrenaline is given tracheally.

Once the patient has received the adrenaline 10 CPR cycles should be carried out while the drug has its effect. During this time a central line can be established if intubation was carried out first, or the patient can be intubated if a central line is in place. Occasionally one or other of these manoeuvres may not be possible; in such cases drug treatment should not be delayed while repeated attempts are made. The available route should be used to administer drugs when they are indicated.

Endotracheal intubation and central venous cannulation are described in Annex A to Chapter 6, and Annex B to Chapter 8, respectively.

12.1.5 Continuing the treatment protocol

The treatment protocol for the diagnosed rhythm should be followed. Ten CPR cycles should be allowed for each drug to have its effect (longer in the case of bretylium tosylate). Adrenaline should be given every 2–3 min during the attempted resuscitation of a patient who has suffered cardiac arrest, whatever their rhythm.

Treatment protocols are shown in detail in Chapter 8.

12.1.6 Reassessment

Throughout resuscitation constant attention should be given to checking that basic life support is still adequate. The rhythm should be monitored for changes, and the functioning of equipment checked. As much history as is available should be gathered.

12.1.7 Post-resuscitation care

Even if adequate spontaneous circulation returns, the airway and ventilation may still require support. Arterial blood gas analysis should be performed urgently. Pharmacological agents may be needed to try to prevent the recurrence of dysrhythmias.

The immediate diagnostic work-up should be commenced as soon as possible, and referral made to the appropriate in-patient facility.

Blood gas interpretation is dealt with in Chapter 5, and post-resuscitation care is discussed in more detail in Chapter 11.

12.2 THE RESUSCITATION TEAM

Team size and the mix of skills within the team will vary widely according to circumstances. Some of the various tasks that may be allocated to team members are:

Airway control and ventilation
External cardiac massage
Defibrillation and rhythm recognition
Establishment of intravascular access
Drug administration
Management of drug and other supplies
Documentation
Liaison
Counselling of relatives

Some of these tasks can be carried out by staff without special skills, and others require staff with appropriate training. If only one member of the team is trained in advanced techniques, then strict adherence to the sequence of events outlined above is essential. If a more skilled team has been assembled then some of the tasks may be addressed concurrently by different team members.

12.3 THE TEAM LEADER

One member of the team must assume the role of team leader. If only one person is a doctor or an advanced cardiac life support provider, the choice of leader is simple. If a team that has more skilled personnel is likely to be present, then the name of the team leader should be clearly stated before the team is on call.

The team leader should be in control of the situation, and should co-ordinate the actions of the team members. The responsibilities of the team leader are:

Directing the team
Checking that assigned tasks are carried out correctly
Ensuring the safety of team members
Assessing the patient
Solving problems
Making the final decision to abandon resuscitation

12.3.1 Direction

Only the team leader should give orders during the resuscitation. This does not exclude other team members from making suggestions, but implies that the final decision rests with the leader.

It is desirable for the team leader to 'stand back' in order to view and direct the whole resuscitation attempt, rather than becoming personally involved in solving individual problems. This is easier if there are a number of skilled people in the team, and very difficult if the leader is also the only skilled person. In the latter case the leader should make deliberate attempts to review the whole resuscitation at regular intervals, in order to check that nothing vital is being missed.

12.3.2 Supervision

The supervision of the team involves ensuring that both basic life support and advanced cardiac life support are being provided correctly, and according to the orders given. Specific points that should be watched for are:

Adequacy of ventilation
Adequacy of external cardiac compression (depth, rate, hand position)
Correct ratio in basic life support
Maintenance of adequate basic life support throughout
Correct and safe defibrillation technique
Assessment of pulse following defibrillation
Correct choice and use of airway adjuncts

Correct ventilator settings
Correct choice and placement of intravascular access
Correct monitor control settings
Correct drugs administered

In general, then, the team leader must be everywhere and check everything.

12.3.3 Safety

The leader also has the responsibility of ensuring that team members are safe. This is particularly important in the out-of-hospital environment, and when potentially hazardous procedures such as defibrillation are being performed.

12.3.4 Patient assessment

Since assessment of the patient is the key to correct decision making, this task is also the responsibility of the team leader. First, the history of the arrest should be established. This can be obtained from nursing and paramedical staff. Pertinent facts are:

Where
When
Witnessed or not
Time to basic life support
Initial rhythm
Time to defibrillation
Special circumstances
Other therapeutic interventions

The past medical history and drug history should be sought. This is more easily obtained for in-patients. In out-of-hospital arrest, relatives may be present or, if not, an urgent retrieval of old hospital notes and a call to the general practitioner can provide invaluable information. Patients often carry prescription cards with them, although their accuracy is sometimes doubtful.

The team leader should also discover whether current signed and dated 'not for resuscitation' orders are in force.

12.3.5 Solving problems

If the patient fails to respond to interventions in an expected manner, then it is the team leader's responsibility to investigate, decide why, and initiate appropriate treatment. This may involve, among other things, reassessing the original diagnosis, recognizing equipment malfunction, or recognizing misplacement of lines or tubes.

The team leader is also responsible for the interpretation of the results of investigations, and initiation of therapy based on them, if appropriate.

12.3.6 Deciding to stop

The decision to stop is always difficult. However, once the diagnosis has been confirmed, the correct treatment protocols applied, other problems such as hypothermia treated, and all relevant history gathered, the team leader should be in a position to do so. It is the team leader's responsibility to make the final decision, but it is usual to discuss this with the rest of the team before stopping.

Practical skill station
Megacode

AIMS

To bring together all the knowledge gained during the course in a simulated arrest situation.

To allow candidates to demonstrate their knowledge of basic life support, dysrhythmia recognition, and treatment protocols gained in theoretical and practical sessions.

To allow candidates to demonstrate proficiency at team leadership.

TEACHING TECHNIQUE

Candidates are nominated as team leader in turn, while the others either critique the performance or act as team members. A scenario is given and the team leader has to organize the resuscitation. This station is carried out using a megacode manikin, which allows practical skills to be carried out as indicated.

TESTING

Candidates are formally tested on their performance at megacode during the examination. Examiners are looking for correct diagnosis and treatment and good team leadership. Errors affecting safety or poor basic life support provision are heavily penalized.

Appendix A
If you don't succeed

Ischaemic heart disease alone causes some 500/100 000 deaths per year in the UK. Many of those affected have no premonitory symptoms, and their first myocardial infarction is fatal. Death is therefore both sudden and unexpected. In such cases relatives and friends of the deceased are totally unprepared.

Failure to resuscitate also presents the medical and nursing staff with emotional burdens, at a time when they are clinically stretched and emotionally vulnerable.

It is often difficult to manage the emotional aspects of critical incidents in the ward or Accident and Emergency department because the situation develops in an unstructured way, over a short period of time. Therefore, a trained member of the resuscitation team must take charge of communication to the relatives as well as their emotional support. This role is filled by a 'relatives' nurse'.

A.1 EMOTIONAL CRISIS: NURSE INTERVENTION

Crisis is an unusual experience, which most people will go through at some time in their life. It is an urgent and stressful situation, which seems overwhelming at the time. However, with the right support from the beginning, most people will come to terms with the experience.

The care of the relatives and friends of the critically ill or dying patient should be seen to be as important as the other tasks in the resuscitation team. The support for distressed relatives begins with their arrival in the ward or Accident and Emergency department, and a trained member of the nursing resuscitation team must be allocated to this task before the patient arrives.

During a crisis, family and friends often gather in the ward or Accident and Emergency department. In the case of sudden death, helpers are often just as devastated as the immediate next of kin. The relatives' nurse needs to be able to act and intervene, being informative as well as compassionate. The care relatives receive in the ward or Accident and Emergency department may well determine their mental well-being during the course of their grief.

The relatives' nurse should accompany the relatives and friends to a private room with suitable facilities available, i.e. telephone, tea-making equipment and toilets. Information useful to the resuscitation team may be gathered from them and this also gives the relatives the opportunity to express or explain how the patient was injured. Likewise, the nurse can inform the relatives of the severity of the patient's present state. By giving them time, a rapport is begun which will be maintained throughout their time in the department.

Explanatory terms such as 'poorly' or 'critical' are meaningless unless accompanied by honest explanation. For example 'cardiac arrest' could be explained as "His heart has stopped beating, he is not breathing and your husband may die". This gives a better account than "Your husband is very ill". Of course, being with already distressed relatives and giving such information is not easy. This may explain why hospital staff tend to give limited information early on in any resuscitative situation. Nonetheless, if relatives are told exactly what is going on, they usually cope much better than if given a modified explanation or, worse still, no explanation at all.

It is an assumption on the part of many hospital staff that relatives may not cope with bad news. Experience has shown that given the facts, most people, though distressed, will deal successfully with the situation. It is when facts are vague that extreme reactions, such as anger and abuse, occur because the relatives feel excluded from the situation and no longer in control. A nurse assigned to the relatives in their crisis can build up a relationship of trust, so that she can act as a link between them and the resuscitation team. This link is very important should the patient die.

The relatives' nurse should also allow a continuous appraisal of the patient's condition to be relayed to the relatives in a structured way. Honest answers to questions, with gentle explanations about what the resuscitation team is attempting, can be given. This nurse can also facilitate arrangements for the family, for example the distressed wife who remembers she has to collect the children from school, and be of further help when other relatives arrive in the ward or department.

A.2 SEEING IS BELIEVING

Should the relatives be allowed to see the patient? This is totally acceptable provided they are accompanied by the relatives' nurse and they are prepared for what they might see. Seeing with their own eyes helps them to come to terms with the event as it is happening. This may be the last time they will see their loved one alive, and so the encounter should not be prevented.

This type of policy can create personal issues for the team members. Nonetheless, these views should not be forced on to others. What is right for one person may be completely wrong for another. Each set of relatives must be allowed to do it their own way while being guided and supported by the nurse.

A.3 THE PHILOSOPHY OF CARING FOR RELATIVES: CULTURAL AND RELIGIOUS ASPECTS

The ward or Accident and Emergency department must have a philosophy for caring for the distressed relatives which is acceptable to their own locality with its various religious and cultural communities. There is no right or wrong way to proceed. Each family is different, but in each case their views and customs must always be respected.

A.4 COMMUNICATION: BREAKING BAD NEWS

There is no standard way of breaking bad news. However, if the relatives are dealt with sensitively and honestly from the very beginning, it can lessen the impact when death has to be announced.

It is unfair to expect the doctor always to break the bad news. The nurse providing support is possibly in a better position to do this should the patient die, since she is the one who has built up a relationship with the relatives. However, it is usual for the team leader to see the bereaved at some time. Before seeing the relatives the facts pertaining to the resuscitation should be gathered together, and some attempt made to remove any blood stains or other marks that may increase distress. All the relatives' questions should be answered in as full a way as possible.

It is at the point of breaking the bad news that medical and nursing staff often feel inadequate. All that can be done is to listen and share the grief as it unfolds. There is no adequate expression which describes our feelings and concern: but sympathy must not be confused with sensitivity.

Words spoken at the time of death will often remain with the relatives forever. Therefore choosing the correct words is important. When breaking the news, care should be taken to avoid using misleading statements. For example, ". . . I'm sorry we lost him" does not describe accurately that someone has died even though that is what is being communicated.

A.5 SAYING 'GOODBYE': VIEWING THE DEAD PERSON

Following the death, the relatives must be given time to allow the information to be absorbed. Every conceivable emotional response is possible in any relative. The relatives' nurse must stay with them to guide them through the next stage of their stay in the ward or Accident and Emergency department.

Shocked and numbed by the news, relatives may leave without saying their 'goodbyes'. Some will regret this in the future, therefore all relatives should be offered the opportunity to see their loved one.

They may never have seen a dead person before and consequently a great deal of fear may be present. The nurse can help displace these anxieties by active encouragement. It is important, especially when death has just occurred, to go with the relatives and let them touch and hold their loved one. If the deceased is a baby then a Moses basket should be available with suggestions given by the nurse as to the holding of their baby.

The relatives must be assured of plenty of time in order to say their 'goodbyes'. There can be no fixed rules and procedures; each family is different and the response must be geared to the particular situation. Their wishes must be respected and if a chaplain is required he should be notified.

If very invasive procedures have taken place, the team may wish to protect the relatives from viewing the body. Unfortunately, though well meant, these actions can lead to problems in the future. The family's fantasy of what the victim might look like could be far worse then the real thing. They have to come to terms with reality. Furthermore, a formal identification of the deceased often has to take place by law. It is better to explain the circumstances and let the relatives decide rather than impose your own perceptions on the family.

It is important that each ward or Accident and Emergency department should be conversant with the local arrangements and have a good working relationship with the local Coroner's officer. In cases of major trauma the deceased person will be deemed to 'belong' to the coroner until the cause of death has been established. This should not interfere with relatives saying their 'goodbyes' and holding and touching their loved ones. Where possible, the coroner's officer should be informed by the team leader and arrangements made for formal identification while the relatives are in the hospital. This will save them from having to return to the mortuary the following day and perhaps compounding their distress.

It is important for the nursing team leader to remember that the deceased's clothing should not be destroyed. This is not only from the point of view of the relatives, but also for legal reasons, as the clothing may be required for forensic evidence.

A.6 FURTHER SUPPORT

Ongoing support is needed for relatives once they leave the ward or Accident and Emergency department. Written information may be required and should be readily available. A useful leaflet is entitled, 'What to do after a death' (Leaflet D.49).

The medical and nursing teams in the community should be informed of the death and clergy may need to be notified. A major asset in this follow-up care is a grief support nurse. This person can act as a link between the hospital and the community it serves.

A.7 STAFF RESPONSE TO DEATH

Following sudden death in the ward or department, it is important to be able to acknowledge the distress among the staff. When actively involved in the resuscitation the team are often performing at their peak. Once the resuscitation has finished, especially if the outcome is death, then time must be taken to unwind. It is the practise in some wards or A/E departments to have an operational debrief to determine if the resuscitation team did everything that was required. It follows that an emotional debrief should take place, albeit informally, with the more experienced members being able to share their feelings with the less experienced. In this way no one person should feel ashamed of feeling sad or inadequate. It is far better to be able to share these feelings rather then 'bottling them up' as the latter can lead to days off duty from sickness or, ultimately, 'burn out'. It takes great courage to say one feels upset, and it takes a non-judgmental team who can share these feelings together so that they are ready to cope with the next critically ill person.

Developing a philosophy of care for the distressed relative and carrying out preventative emotional debriefing for all staff members reduces the future need for counselling, therapy and psychiatric intervention. Prevention is better than cure, and more cost-effective!

A.8 THE ROLE OF THE CORONER

In most cases of sudden death, the coroner will make arrangements for the deceased to be removed for formal examination. Following this, he is obliged by law to hold an inquest if death cannot be attributable to natural causes. A post mortem (PM) may or may not precede an inquest, but if one is ordered by the coroner, the person in possession of the body has no choice but to agree. The PM is usually carried out by an independent pathologist appointed by the coroner but interested parties have a right to be represented at this examination by a medical practitioner.

A.8.1 Inquests

These meetings allow the interested parties to ask questions of the witnesses called by the coroner. They are also open to the public and press.

It is the coroner's officer who is responsible for preparing the evidence and organizing the inquest proceedings and, to this end, is responsible for assembling all the statements and evidence.

Members of resuscitation teams are likely to be involved in an inquest at some stage of their careers. Evidence is usually given orally, with the coroner initially taking the witness through their statement, before they are cross-examined.

A.9 HELP GROUPS

All of these help groups have local contacts. The national offices will provide helpful leaflets and further information.

CRUSE (Bereavement care)
126 Sheen Road
Richmond
Surrey
TW9 IUR
Tel. 081 940 4818

The Compassionate Friends (An international organization of bereaved parents)
6 Denmark Street
Bristol
BS1 5DQ
Tel. 0272 292 778

The Foundation for the Study of Infant Deaths
35 Belgrave Square
London
SWIX 8PS
Tel. 071 235 0965

Stillbirth and Neonatal Death Society (SANDS)
28 Portland Place
London
W1N 4DE
Tel. 071 436 5881

The Samaritans (24-hour support for the despairing)
Local branches in most towns in the UK

REFERENCES AND FURTHER READING

Awooner-Renner, S. (1991) I desperately need to see my son. *Br. Med. J.*, **302**, 356.

Finlay, I. and Dallimore, D. (1991) Your child is dead. *Br. Med. J.*, **302**, 1524.

Lake, A. (1987) *Living with Grief.* Heinemann, London.

McLauchlan, C. (1990) Handling distressed relatives and breaking bad news. In *ABC of Major Trauma*, edited by D. Skinner, P. Driscoll and R. Earlam. *Br. Med. J.*, **301**, 1145.

Werthaimer, A. (1991) *A Special Scar.* Routledge, London

Woodward, S., Pope, A. and Robson, W. (1985) Bereavement counselling after sudden infant death. *Br. Med. J.*, **290**, 363.

Worden, J. (1983) *Grief Counselling and Grief Therapy.* Tavistock, London.

Yates, D., Ellison, G. and McGuiness, S. (1990) Care of the suddenly bereaved. *Br. Med. J.*, **301**, 29.

Appendix B
Ethical and legal considerations in resuscitation

This article by Dr Patrick Dando was first published as 'Medico-Legal Problems Associated with Resuscitation' in the *Journal of the Medical Defence Union*, Volume 8, Numbers 1 and 2, 1992. It is reproduced here with kind permission of the Medical Defence Union and Dr Patrick Dando. All rights reserved.

The provision of resuscitation to a collapsed and perhaps unconscious patient is professionally demanding. As in any branch of medicine, the practitioner (any member of a resuscitation team) having taken on the duty of care to a patient is expected to provide a reasonable standard of treatment. Medical negligence may be alleged if there is a breach of that duty leading to a foreseeable injury to the patient for which the patient may claim compensation.

B.1 LEGAL BACKGROUND

Such an action is brought under the civil law of tort (meaning wrongdoing) under which a patient is compensated for injuries resulting from negligence. It is not appropriate to define absolute standards of care required from practitioners but, in the event of a claim of medical negligence, experts in the relevant field give opinions based on the circumstances of the case in the light of accepted standards at the time the events occurred. This follows the test of Mr Justice McNair who gave judgement in 1957 in the case of Bolam v Friern Hospital Management Committee and stated:

> "The test is the standard of the ordinary skilled man exercising and professing to have that special skill. A man need not possess the highest expert skill at the risk of being found negligent. It is well-established law that it is sufficient if he exercises the ordinary skill of an ordinary man exercising that particular art."[1]

The jury were directed by Mr Justice McNair: "A doctor is not negligent, if he is acting in accordance with a practice accepted as proper by a responsible body of medical men skilled in that particular art, merely because there is a body of such opinion that takes a contrary view."[2]

A medical negligence action will not be successful if the injury results from the normal risks associated with that particular branch of care, nor is a practitioner expected to bring an exceptional level of skill but must apply the ordinary level possessed by practitioners working in the same specialty. It is understood that there may be more than one acceptable method of treatment.

It may be very difficult for the experts advising in a medical negligence action concerning resuscitation to distinguish between an injury caused by the illness which led to a patient's collapse and one which might have been caused by resuscitation. The experts called by the defendant and the plaintiff may hold different opinions. The issue may have to be settled at trial where a judge, on the balance of probabilities, will make a decision after considering the evidence.

During resuscitation, judgements may have to be made quickly concerning diagnosis and treatment. An error of judgement may not necessarily be negligent.

At the House of Lords in 1981, Lord Fraser, hearing the appeal in Whitehouse v Jordan, said: "Merely to describe something as an error of judgement tells us nothing about whether it is negligent or not. The true position is that an error of judgement may, or may not, be negligent; it depends on the nature of the error. If it is one that would not have been made by a reasonably competent professional man professing to have the standard and type of skill that the defendant held himself out as having, and acting with ordinary care, then it is negligent. If, on the other hand, it is an error that a man, acting with ordinary care, might have made, then it is not negligence."[3]

Training and supervised practice in the techniques and complexities of resuscitation are essential. Following proper instruction and supervised practice, self-audit is a great aid to improving technique. It is essential that a practitioner keeps up to date with new developments in resuscitation. Those responsible for supervising training must satisfy themselves of an individual's capacity to work in the field and ensure that any protocols are revised as new developments become part of standard procedures.

Earlier, in the Appeal Court, Donaldson L J had stated: "If a doctor fails to exercise the skill which he has or claims to have, he is in breach of his duty of care. He is negligent."[4]

Inexperience cannot be a defence to an action of medical negligence. Glidewell L J in Wilsher v Essex Area Health Authority 1987 said ". . . the inexperienced doctor called upon to exercise a specialist skill will, as part of that skill, seek the advice and help of his superiors when he does or may need it. If he does seek such help, he will often have satisfied the test, even though he may himself have made a mistake."[5]

This does imply that the inexperienced practitioner can recognize when help is needed. In an emergency specialist help may not be available immediately but should be sought when possible.

Practitioners who are not medically qualified must be particularly careful not to exceed the skills with which they have been accredited. Nor should they accept delegation of such responsibilities from their employers until they are satisfied in their own minds of their competence.

A person who unexpectedly comes across the scene of an accident has no absolute duty in British law to act positively for the benefit of others but most people would consider it an ethical duty, and the General Medical Council (GMC) states that the public is entitled to expect a registered medical practitioner to provide 'appropriate and prompt action upon evidence suggesting the existence of a condition requiring urgent medical intervention'.[6] GPs as part of their terms of service are expected to provide emergency treatment to any person who requires it within their practice area.[7] A practitioner with special skills in resuscitation who offers assistance takes on a duty of care and must exercise it within the constraints imposed by the prevailing circumstances.

Since the introduction of NHS indemnity on 1 January 1990 doctors who work for a health authority are indemnified by their employer, which is vicariously liable for the acts of its employees and has to meet the costs for damages and legal expenses of a successful claim from its own budget. (GPs and doctors who treat patients privately make their own arrangements for professional indemnity through one of the medical defence organizations). NHS indemnity does not cover health authority employees who provide voluntary professional assistance at accidents and disasters outside of their employment. Many doctors in the hospital and community services join a medical defence organization which can provide indemnity for 'Good Samaritan' acts as one of the benefits of membership.

B.2 POTENTIAL PITFALLS IN RESUSCITATION

A patient's condition may deteriorate rapidly, without warning and there is an obligation to identify any patient who is critically ill within an A&E or other department, and ensure that the patient is appropriately observed and resuscitation given with expedition if necessary.

A patient's collapse should be brought to the urgent attention of the resuscitation team who have to react immediately. The need for resuscitation may have occurred in the comparative luxury of a fully equipped and staffed resuscitation room or at a less convenient site, such as a hospital car park, a river bank or the patient's workplace or home. In these circumstances the resuscitation team must travel and take their equipment with them. Despite the urgency it is most important that the team does no harm to the patient, to others or to themselves. On arrival at the scene care is necessary to check for electrical, chemical and other hazards, which could have been responsible for the collapse and may present a danger to the rescuers. Appropriate action must be taken to eliminate such a danger.

With very limited exceptions a person suffering from an illness or an injury does not have to submit to examination or treatment if he refuses. However, if resuscitation is necessary the patient will usually be unconscious and unable to give consent. In an emergency the doctor should proceed and the treatment provided without specific consent must not be more extensive than is necessary to cope with the immediate emergency. If it is known that the patient would object to a treatment – an example would be a Jehovah's Witness who had clearly indicated the wish not to receive any blood product – that wish must be taken into consideration.

Clearing the airway from obstruction by secretions, vomit or foreign bodies, as well as its protection and maintenance is fundamental to resuscitation. While establishing an airway, dentures should be removed and practitioners should take as much care as possible of the teeth during intubation. If a tooth is dislodged, it should be located and if it is not found this fact should be recorded and at a later date a chest X-ray can be taken to exclude the possibility of aspiration. The usual anaesthetic precautions should be taken to ensure that an endotracheal tube is appropriately sited and the possibility of oesophageal intubation is excluded. Oesophageal intubation is not necessarily negligent but on most occasions failure to detect it is. If there is inadequate respiratory effort, time should not be wasted trying a difficult intubation when other means of artificial ventilation are available.

Drugs and fluids may need to be given intravenously and care must be taken to ensure that the correct ampoule or bottle has been selected. A well-functioning intravenous line is invaluable and should be established as soon as possible. Certain agents, especially sodium bicarbonate, may act as an irritant if they extravasate and care should be taken to ensure that an intravenous line is functioning properly and has not been sited in an artery. It should be replaced if there are any doubts. When intravenous fluids are being given, care should be taken that they do not run through unnoticed.

Electrical defibrillation should be performed by somebody trained in its use and care must be taken that none of the resuscitators are in physical contact with the patient at the time of application of the electrodes. The patient's condition may warrant the insertion of a central venous pressure line, a hazard being that this may, albeit rarely, provoke a pneumothorax. This is not usually considered negligent, but the possibility should be borne in mind and excluded by a chest X-ray if necessary. The route selected by the doctor for the insertion of the CVP line should be that with which he is most familiar.

The unconscious patient cannot complain of pain and care must be taken that limbs are not placed in unsuitable positions with the risk of damage by pressure to peripheral blood supply or peripheral nerves or over-stretching of the brachial plexus. The head and particularly the eyes should be protected against inadvertent trauma.

In the course of resuscitation the practitioners will attempt to glean information, which is often limited, to establish a diagnosis and to provide appropriate treatment. On occasion the patient will carry a card or a 'medic alert' bracelet giving details of medication, allergies or of an illness, which can be extremely helpful. The patient may be carrying bottles of medication or a repeat prescription card from his GP which can be helpful and should be looked for, though it might need to be followed up in due course by a telephone call. Relatives or friends accompanying the patient can be a source of invaluable information and attempts should be made to identify and question them.

During resuscitation blood and other samples may be taken for urgent analysis and it is most important that containers and request forms are accurately labelled. If the patient's name is not known a reference number might be used. The specimens should be taken to the laboratory where staff should be informed that the results are required urgently. The requesting doctor is responsible for ensuring that the result is received and acted on appropriately.

It is vital to keep clear and concise records to provide detailed information to those who subsequently take on care of a patient. In the event of a medical negligence claim, such records will also provide proof of the facts of the case at some distant time. It is said that without a record there is no defence. The record should be made as soon as practicable and in some circumstances it is possible to designate one member of staff as the 'recorder' while resuscitation is continuing. It should contain relevant information on the observations made, drugs given with their dosage and timing, and details of the strength and timing of defibrillation. The record must be signed, dated, timed and be legible. It should be stored carefully together with any ECG tracing or pathology reports until they can be placed in the patient's file.

The patient who is successfully resuscitated will usually be transferred to an ITU and responsibility rests with the resuscitation team to pass on all relevant information. If possible this should be done orally and should be supplemented with a written record.

On other occasions the patient is not successfully resuscitated and close relatives will have to be informed. If a relative is near at hand, a private place must be found to explain what has happened. It is a difficult task which will usually be undertaken by a senior member of the team. If there is a request to see the body before it is moved, it may be possible to remove the various lines and tubes and make the body suitable to be seen; unless it is likely that the pathologist (or coroner) would wish them to remain *in situ* or has earlier made it clear that he would always wish for them to be left in place. The patient's property should be itemized and given to a near relative, who should be requested to sign a receipt, or it can be given to a hospital administrator for safe keeping. On occasions the patient may not have been identified and assistance from the police may be required.

Sometimes it is possible for a medical practitioner to provide a death certificate if he has been in attendance during the patient's last illness. However, in every case of violent or unnatural death or sudden death, the cause of which is unknown, including a death following an accident, the doctor should notify the coroner immediately and will often be asked to provide a statement to the coroner's officer concerning the circumstances of the case.

On a few occasions a medical mishap may have caused a patient's collapse or one might have occurred during resuscitation. In that event it may be appropriate for the patient or the immediate relatives to be told of the facts by a senior medical member of the team. It is advisable to avoid speculation or comment on the actions of others. The simple courtesy of a sincere and honest apology may be necessary in certain circumstances.

The suddenness of a patient's collapse may be regarded as newsworthy by the public but the duty of confidentiality owed to a patient must be respected even after the patient's death. The media can be very insistent and sometimes it may be possible to answer queries by issuing a statement through the health authority's administration.

After resuscitation non-disposable equipment must be sterilized to prevent the risk of cross-infection. The usual precautions should be taken to avoid self-contamination by blood and other biological products. Used needles and other sharps should not be resheathed, risking self-inoculation, but placed into a sharps bin for later incineration. Hepatitis B immunization should be considered by any practitioner involved in resuscitation.

It is important that all equipment is checked regularly to ensure that it is functioning properly and that drugs have not become time-expired. The Consumer Protection Act 1987 requires a producer to ensure that a product is up to standard and fit for the intended purpose. If a patient suffers damage from a defect in a piece of equipment during the course of treatment, the liability rests with the producer who may escape that liability if it can be shown that the equipment was not maintained or calibrated or used in accordance with the instructions. The records for servicing must be kept for 11 years and are essential if liability is to be passed on to the producer in the event of the product being in some way faulty.

B.3 CONCLUSION

Through the competent application of their expertise the resuscitation team may draw upon the satisfaction of a job well done. If a patient dies, his relatives and friends will often appreciate that considerable efforts have been made in sometimes very adverse conditions.

REFERENCES

1. [1957] 2 ALL ER 118 at 121.
2. [1957] 2 ALL ER 118.
3. [1981] 1 ALL ER 267 at 281.
4. [1980] 1 ALL ER 650 at 662.
5. [1986] 3 ALL ER 801 at 831.
6. Professional Conduct & Discipline: Fitness to Practise. GMC. February 1991: 10.
7. Terms of Service for Doctors in General Practice, February 1991, 4 (1) (h).

Appendix C
The theory of acid–base balance

C.1 ACID

As explained in chapter 5, an acid is a substance which dissociates in aqueous solution to produce a hydrogen ion (H^+) and its conjugate base. For example, hydrogen chloride dissociates in water to give hydrochloric acid:

$$HCl \rightleftharpoons H^+ + Cl^-$$

In this case Cl^- is the conjugate base. This dissociation can be written in general terms as:

$$[HB] \rightleftharpoons [H^+] + [B^-]$$

where the square brackets indicate concentrations.

Eventually the rate of reaction from left to right equals the rate of reaction from right to left. At this stage, the concentrations of the acid, base and hydrogen ion no longer change with time, i.e the amount of HB dissociating equals the amount of H^+ and B^- recombining. The reaction is then said to be at equilibrium.

For a strong acid, equilibrium is reached when most of the acid has dissociated and the balance of the equation lies mainly to the right. A weak acid, on the other hand, does not dissociate so readily and, at equilibrium, the balance of the equation lies mainly to the left. Most acids within the body are weak.

C.1.1 Acid dissociation constants and pK_a

Once equilibrium has been reached, the products of the concentrations of the reactants on one side of the equation are proportional to those on the other. This can be expressed as:

$$[HB] \; \alpha \; [H^+][B^-]$$

The strength of an acid, i.e. the degree to which it will dissociate, can therefore be expressed as the constant that describes the proportion of dissociation that occurs. This is called the acid dissociation constant, K_a.

$$K_a[HB] = [H^+][B^-]$$

A simple rearrangement of the equation above gives the following expression for K_a:

$$K_a = \frac{[H^+][B^-]}{[HB]}$$

The higher the value of K_a, the stronger the acid. Thus a strong acid, which is virtually completely dissociated, has a very large value for its acid dissociation constant, while a weak acid, which is only partially dissociated, has a small value.

Because the dissociation constants of relatively weak acids are so small, they are most conveniently expressed logarithmically. For ease of use the inverse of K_a is used since this ensures that values are positive:

$$pK_a = \log_{10}\frac{1}{K_a}$$

Since division is achieved by subtraction of logarithms, an alternative expression for the equation above is:

$$pK_a = \log_{10}1 - \log_{10}[K_a]$$

and, as $\log_{10}1$ is 0, this means that:

$$pK_a = -\log_{10}K_a$$

The higher the value of pK_a, the weaker the acid.

C.1.2 pH

Since hydrogen ion concentrations are so small, acid–base status is also described using an inverse logarithmic scale. This scale has the advantage of being able to express all H^+ concentrations as simple positive numbers. pH is defined as:

$$pH = \log_{10}\frac{1}{[H^+]}$$

where $[H^+]$ represents the hydrogen ion concentration.

For the reasons described for pK_a above, an alternative expression for this is:

$$pH = -\log_{10}[H^+]$$

pH can therefore be defined as the negative of the logarithm to the base 10 of the hydrogen ion concentration.

To illustrate this, consider a hydrogen ion concentration of 10^{-8}

(0.000 000 01 or one hundred millionth) mol/l. The pH value is derived as follows:

$$pH = -\log_{10}10^{-8}$$
$$\log_{10}10^{-8} = -8$$

therefore

$$pH = -(-8)$$

or

$$pH = 8$$

Recently there has been a move back towards expressing the acidity of a solution as its actual hydrogen ion concentration. Unlike the logarithmic pH scale, the $[H^+]$ of a solution increases linearly as acidity increases. The normal plasma $[H^+]$ is about 40 nmol/l [a nanomole (nmol) is 0.000 000 001 of a molar concentration].

C.1.3 Henderson's equation

The general equation for acid dissociation shown at the beginning of this appendix can be rearranged in terms of the hydrogen ion concentration as shown below:

$$[H^+] = K_a\frac{[HB]}{[B^-]}$$

This is known as the Henderson equation and it shows that acidity, the hydrogen ion concentration, depends on the ratio of the acid to its conjugate base, and not on the absolute value of either.

C.1.3.1 Henderson–Hasselbalch equation

Inverting the equation above results in:

$$\frac{1}{[H^+]} = \frac{[B^-]}{K_a[HB]}$$

This new expression for the inverse hydrogen ion concentration can be used to derive a new expression for pH:

$$pH = \log_{10}\frac{1}{[H^+]} = \log_{10}\frac{[B^-]}{k_a[HB]}$$

Since multiplication is achieved by addition of logarithms, this new expression can be written as:

$$pH = \log_{10}\frac{1}{K_a} + \log_{10}\frac{[B^-]}{[HB]}$$

Substituting pK_a results in the equation below:

$$pH = pK_a + \log_{10}\frac{[B^-]}{[HB]}$$

This is known as the Henderson–Hasselbalch equation and shows how pH and pK_a values are linked.

If carbonic acid is entered into the Henderson–Hasselbalch equation the result is:

$$[H^+] = K\frac{[H_2CO_3]}{[HCO_3^-]}$$

The concentration of carbonic acid ($[H_2CO_3]$) is difficult to measure, but it can be replaced with the partial pressure of CO_2 dissolved in 100mls of arterial plasma ($PaCO_2$), multiplied by its solubility coefficient in blood (α):

$$[H^+] = K\frac{\alpha PaCO_2}{[HCO_3^-]}$$

This equation demonstrates that the acidity or pH of blood depends on the ratio of the dissolved carbon dioxide to the bicarbonate concentration, rather than on their absolute values. $PaCO_2$, in turn, is dependant on the balance between the production of CO_2 and its elimination by alveolar ventilation.

Typical values are $[HCO_3^-]$ = 24 mmol/l, $PaCO_2$ = 5.3 kPa, solubility coefficient = 0.225 mmol/l/Kpa, and pK_a = 6.1. Therefore:

$$pH = 6.1 + \log\frac{24}{0.225 \times 5.3}$$

$$pH = 6.1 + \log 20$$

$$pH = 6.1 + 1.3 \therefore pH = 7.4$$

C.2 BUFFERS

The efficiency of a buffer is determined by its pK_a value. At this point it has equal potential to take up or donate H^+ ions.

	pK_a
Protein	= 7.0
Haemoglobin	= 7.4
Phosphate	= 6.8
Carbonic acid	= 6.1

The first three pK_a levels are similar to the normal pH levels in their respective environments and so these buffers will be working at near maximum efficiency.

In contrast, the carbonic acid–bicarbonate system is not working in an optimum pH environment. This disadvantage is overcome by it being present in large quantities in the extracellular fluid, and by its ability to eliminate the acid load by ventilation. This latter point enables carbonic acid to link ventilation with metabolic H^+ production.

C.3 KIDNEYS

Hydrogen ions are removed in the kidney by combination with monohydrogen phosphate (HPO_4^{2-}) to form dihydrogen phosphate ($H_2PO_4^-$), by production of ammonium ions (NH_4^+) from glutamine, by exchange with sodium ions and by direct secretion (Figure C.1).

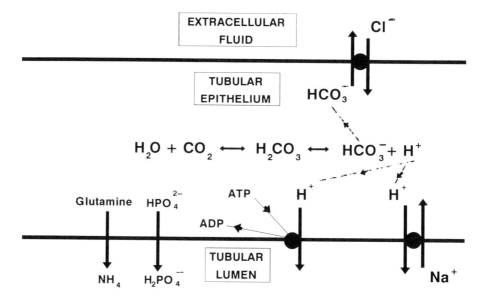

Fig. C.1 Renal mechanisms

In the renal tubule, hydrogen ions react with filtered bicarbonate to form water and CO_2. The latter diffuses rapidly into the renal tubular cell where carbonic anhydrase catalyses the formation of carbonic acid and hence bicarbonate and hydrogen ion. The former is absorbed into the extracellular fluid and the latter is excreted into the tubular lumen.

C.4 ACIDOSIS AND ALKALOSIS

C.4.1 Simple disturbances

These are due to only one disturbance in the acid–base system.

C.4.1.1 Metabolic acidosis

With a metabolic acidosis, there is a marked change in the plasma bicarbonate concentration (E in Figure C.2).

For example, if 4 mmols of a strong acid is added to a litre of a buffer system designed to imitate plasma with a bicarbonate of 24 mmol and a constant PCO_2 of 5.3 kPa, carbonic acid is produced. This dissociates with a loss of 4 mmol of CO_2 via the lungs and a reduction in bicarbonate of 4 mmols:

$$H^+ + HCO_3^- \rightarrow H_2CO_3 \rightarrow HCO_3^- + CO_2 \uparrow + H_2O$$

in mmol/l:

$$4 + 24 \rightarrow H_2CO_3 \rightarrow 20 + 4 + 4$$

For practical purposes, in an acute metabolic acidosis the fall in bicarbonate equals the amount of acid added.

In the ensuing hours and days the kidneys will excrete the excess hydrogen ions and regenerate bicarbonate so that a near normal acid–base balance is restored.

C.4.1.2 Respiratory acidosis

It is important to realise that the carbonic acid buffer system does not buffer respiratory acid production – an acid cannot react with its own salt. Instead other buffers are used.

In comparison to the large changes seen in metabolic acidosis, there is little change in the bicarbonate concentration in the acute phase of respiratory acidosis. However, the ratio between bicarbonate and carbonic acid alters so that it becomes less than 20:1.

As an example, consider the doubling of the normal $PaCO_2$ to 10.6 kPa, with a consequent increase in dissolved CO_2 from 1.2 to 2.4 mmol/l. If there was no change in the bicarbonate, the hydrogen ion concentration would increase from 40 nmol/l to 80 nmol/l and the pH would fall to 7.1. However, the formation of this extra $[H^+]$ only leads to an equivalent amount of HCO_3^- with the new $[HCO_3^-]$ being 24.00004 mmol/l:

$$H_2O + CO_2 + NaHCO_3 \rightleftharpoons H^+ + HCO_3^- + NaHCO_3$$

in mmol/l:

$$2.4 + 24 \rightleftharpoons 0.00004 + 0.00004 + 24$$

For all practical purposes, in the acute phase of a respiratory acidosis, the plasma bicarbonate concentration remains constant (C in Figure C.2).

The bicarbonate concentration does increase with time following renal (chronic) compensation (D in Figure C.2).

C.4.1.3 Metabolic alkalosis

This can follow nasogastric suction, vomiting and excessive bicarbonate administration. Alveolar hypoventilation may lead to compensatory respiratory acidosis.

C.4.1.4 Respiratory alkalosis

This follows a mismatch between CO_2 production and alveolar ventilation leading to a decreased $PaCO_2$. Early compensation (15 min) (A in Figure C.2) is by shift of hydrogen, chloride and lactate ions from the intracellular to extracellular compartment. A further compensatory metabolic acidosis occurs with reduction in plasma bicarbonate. This is relatively slow to occur.

As the kidneys adjust there is an increase in hydrogen ion retention and a decrease in bicarbonate reabsorption. This helps restore the pH towards normal (B in Figure C.2).

Interpretation of acid–base data may be aided by a diagrammatic representation such as Figure C.2. This has been adapted from the paper by Flenley.

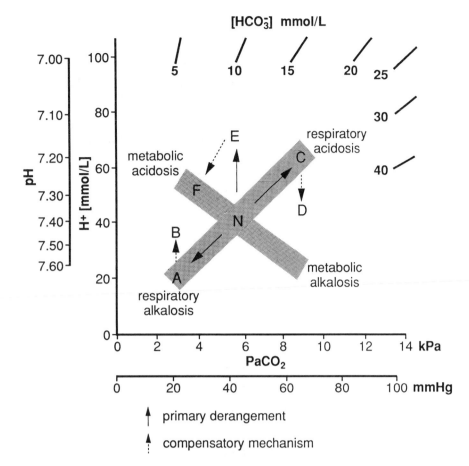

**Fig. C.2
Flenley diagram**

[HCO₃] mmol/L

primary derangement

compensatory mechanism

C.4.2 Mixed disturbances

These involve either two disturbances to the acid–base system or one abnormality with medical attempts to correct it. In these cases, the acid–base picture may well lie outside the normal compensatory bands indicated in Figure C.2.

C.4.3 The plasma anion gap

This gives further information about the state of the acid–base balance of the patient. It is defined as:

$$[Na^+ + K^+] - [HCO_3^- + Cl^-]$$

and it is due to the presence of unmeasured anions such as phosphate, sulphate and albumin. The commonly accepted normal value is 8–16 mmol/l.

The gap allows differentiation of the less common acidosis which have a normal value, from the more common acidosis which have a high value:

C.4.3.1 Acidosis with an increased anion gap

This is commonly due to an elevation in the plasma acids which are not measured in the equation. These are usually organic in nature and the causes include:

Ketoacidosis	Diabetes mellitus Alcoholism Starvation
Lactic Acidosis	Poor tissue perfusion Phenformin treatment Severe alkalaemia
Renal failure	Retention of acid metabolites
Poisoning	Salicylates Ethylene glycol Methanol

A useful mneumonic is 'mudsleep' = methanol, uraemia, diabetic ketoacidosis, salicylic acid, lactic acidosis, ethylene glycol, ethanol and paraldehyde.

C.4.3.2 Acidosis with a normal anion gap

In these cases there is a decrease in the plasma bicarbonate but retention of chloride. The causes include:

Failure of renal acidification	Renal tubular acidosis Acetazolamide
Bicarbonate loss from the gut	Diarrhoea Small bowel fistula Ureterosigmoidostomy

Index